GANDHI'S
JOHANNESBURG

GANDHI'S
JOHANNESBURG

Birthplace of Satyagraha

ERIC ITZKIN

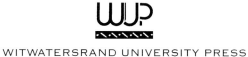

WITWATERSRAND UNIVERSITY PRESS

in association with

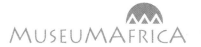

FRANK CONNOCK PUBLICATION No 4

Witwatersrand University Press
1 Jan Smuts Avenue
2001 Johannesburg
South Africa

ISBN 1 86814 361 9

First published in 2000

Typesetting and Cover Design: Sue Sandrock
Printed and bound by Creda Communications, Cape Town

ACKNOWLEDGEMENTS

My heartfelt thanks go to David Saks for his valuable research and advice. I have also benefited greatly from unpublished research and comments from Professor James Hunt. As usual, Alan Buff was a mine of information. Thanks are also due to E S Reddy and Elsabé Brink.

The Indian Council for Cultural Relations, New Delhi, funded the research. The project to document Gandhi sites in the Johannesburg area was initiated by Mr S R Tayal, the Consul General for India in South Africa from 1996 to 1998. Assistance from Mr N G Patel and the Gandhi Centenary Council helped bring the work to completion.

Many thanks to my colleagues at MuseuMAfricA: to Hilary Bruce for her support; Sandra de Wet for digital imaging; and Carolina Geldenhuys for help with the maps.

Images from MuseuMAfricA's collections were supplemented by: Johannesburg Metropolitan Library Services, the Indian Cultural Centre (Johannesburg), *The Star*, Stucke Harrison Archives, Sally Gaule and Ramy Pillay.

Thanks to my wife, Ayesha, for pointing me eastwards. And in memory of my father, Max Itzkin, supporter of the Indian passive resistance of 1946.

At weekends Gandhi and a small party of us would go for a picnic to some beauty spot in the Transvaal or bathe in the lake at Rosherville on the East Rand. These were happy gatherings and Gandhi was a most enthusiastic participator in all the fun. ... People who only got to know Gandhi as an old man will find it hard to realise that he was once a young man, a little over thirty, bright and cheerful and full of the joy of life.

Albert West

Up to the year 1906 I simply relied on appeal to reason. I was a very industrious reformer. ... But I found that reason failed to produce an impression when the critical moment arrived in South Africa. My people were excited – even a worm can and does turn – and there was talk of wreaking vengeance. I had then to choose between allying myself to violence or finding out some other method of meeting the crisis and stopping the rot, and it came to me that we should refuse to obey legislation that was degrading and let them put us in jail if they liked. Thus came into being the moral equivalent of war.

Mohandas Gandhi

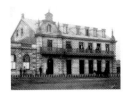

CONTENTS

FOREWORD

MOHANDAS KARAMCHAND GANDHI was twenty-four years old when he boarded the train in Durban bound for the Transvaal. He had not intended to leave the train anywhere en route, but he did so in Pietermaritzburg and the story of his unexpected interlude on the Pietermaritzburg railway platform belongs to the genre of epic transformations,* though the full story of the transformed months and years that followed is still inadequately known.

From 1893 to 1914 Gandhi waged battle after brave battle against racial discrimination. Though much of that time was spent in Durban and in the Phoenix Settlement which he established outside Durban, a good deal was also spent in the Transvaal – in Pretoria, Johannesburg and on the fecund acreage of Tolstoy Farm near that city where, under his direct attention, fruit and passive resistance grew.

It was in these places that Gandhi moved – and helped others move – into the domain of future history. Lawyer, activist, pamphleteer, journalist, author, farmer, householder, passive resister, prisoner and negotiator, he made lifelong friends there and found causes and affiliations that were to last him a lifetime.

In various homes, offices, legal chambers, courts and in the public spaces in which he was seen, he came to be understood, respected, trusted and loved. But such were the complexities of his undertaking, and such his sense of fair play, that he was also spurned, misunderstood, reviled and attacked – verbally and even physically.

Gandhi emerged from each of those experiences with greater strength and determination to meet the challenges that lay in the future. And it was here, in the ebb and flow of the outer struggle, that he came to terms with some of his own inner conflicts, in the resolution of which his wife Kasturba played a singularly important and defining role.

Gandhi was forty-six when he left South Africa. Natal and the Transvaal, the scenes of brave resistances and trusting accords, had already made him, after Dadabhai Naoroji, the best known Indian outside India.

This carefully researched book takes the reader to those paths and sites in and near Johannesburg where the alchemised Gandhi worked and gave practical shape to his new-found vision. But the book also does more. It suggests coordinates for the kind of principled linkages that Gandhi would have wanted us to seek in our present times. For, if great destinations have been reached in countries like South Africa and India, new journeys that lie further ahead are also coming sharply to view.

Gopalkrishna Gandhi
High Commissioner for India in South Africa
1997-1998

---

* Gandhi's life was forever changed on Pietermaritzburg Station in 1893. Newly arrived in South Africa, he was thrown off the train for insisting on his right to travel first class. When the conductor ordered him to transfer from a 'whites only' section to a third-class compartment, he refused. Gandhi himself later traced the genesis of his resolve to oppose injustice to the cold night spent in the waiting room.

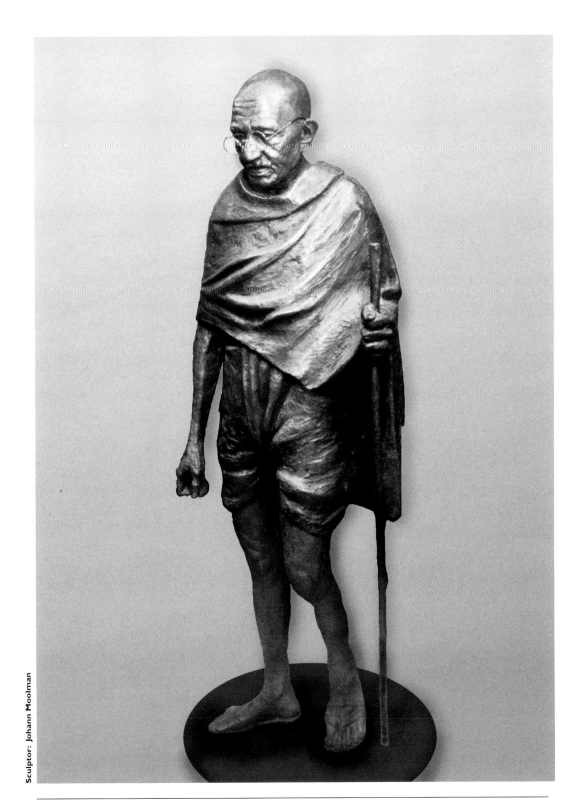

Life-size statue of Mahatma Gandhi at the new Gandhi Hall in Lenasia

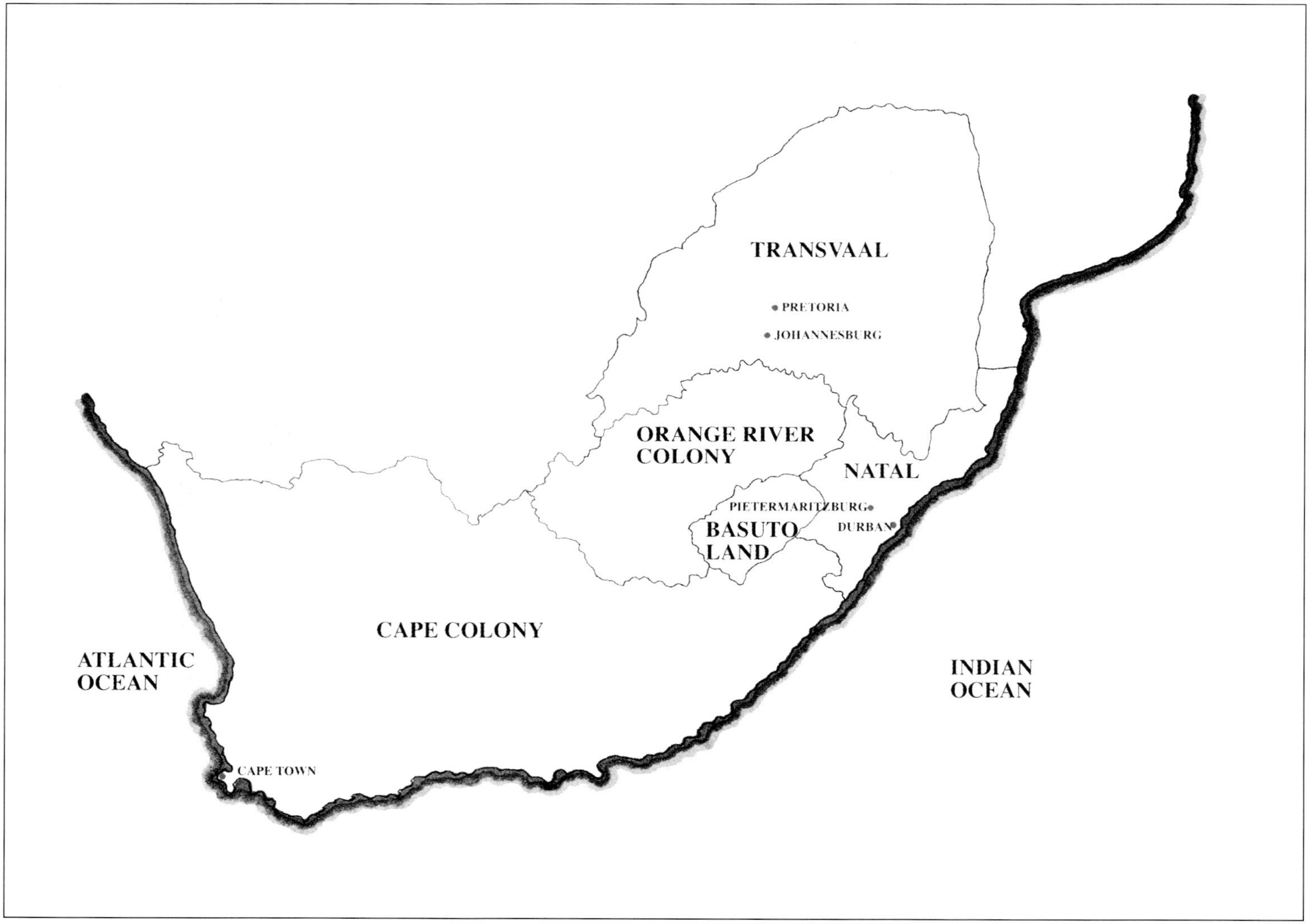

TRANSVAAL

● PRETORIA

● JOHANNESBURG

ORANGE RIVER
COLONY

NATAL

PIETERMARITZBURG ●

DURBAN ●

BASUTO
LAND

CAPE COLONY

CAPE TOWN

ATLANTIC
OCEAN

INDIAN
OCEAN

South Africa, 1900

INTRODUCTION

Eric Itzkin

None of us knew what name to give to our movement. I then used the term passive resistance in describing it. I did not quite understand the implications of passive resistance as I called it. I only knew that some new principle had come into being.

Mohandas Gandhi

FROM THE bustling young mining town of Johannesburg came ideals of peaceful struggle which spread across the world. First formulated by Mohandas Gandhi (1869-1948) in the early 1900s, the philosophy of Satyagraha inspired popular struggles throughout the twentieth century and hastened the end of colonial empires internationally.

Gandhi first rose to prominence in South Africa and later made his mark in India where his concept of passive resistance helped shape the protest movements that led to the collapse of the British Raj and the achievement of independence.

While it is chiefly for his work in India that Gandhi came to be revered by many millions of people, in his time and afterwards, the path that took him to the head of India's independence movement leads back to his early formative years in South Africa. Experiences gathered during his time there, especially his political baptism in Johannesburg, prepared Gandhi for the epic struggles that crowned the closing decades of his life in India.

When he arrived in South Africa in 1893 there was little about him to suggest the makings of a world figure. At the age of twenty-four, he was shy and lacking in confidence. His academic record was undistinguished and, after he qualified as barrister in London in 1891, his legal career in India was bitterly disappointing. His first brief, from a poor woman called Mamibai, was disastrous. As he rose to cross examine a witness, he was struck with stage fright and collapsed in his chair. During the remaining months in India Gandhi never entered a court again.

An offer of work in South Africa brought the promise of a new start. The contract was to assist Dada Abdullah, a wealthy businessman based in Durban, in a lawsuit against a cousin in Johannesburg. Though Gandhi soon settled the dispute with a compromise that satisfied both parties, his sojourn in South Africa was to last for twenty-one years, broken only by brief interludes in England and India.

The success he achieved in the Dada Abdullah case enhanced Gandhi's prestige and prompted Indian merchants in Durban to engage his services. While running his legal practice in Durban Gandhi made early forays into politics. As a lawyer and fledgling politician he fought against the restrictive laws applied to Indians, although mounting any sustained challenge to discrimination was still beyond him.

In 1902, Gandhi left for India where he intended to establish a legal practice in Bombay but, faithful to his pledge that he would come back to South Africa if the Indian community there needed him, he returned to represent Indians who were barred from entering the Transvaal.

The many Indian refugees who left the Transvaal during the Anglo-Boer War of 1899-1902 were prevented from returning to their homes and businesses once the war was over. Indians who had remained in the Transvaal also found that their position had worsened after the British victory. The new British officials revived the anti-Indian laws of their Boer predecessors and enforced them with a vengeance. Indians could not own fixed property, live outside segregated locations, or trade outside designated bazaars. Realising the gravity of the situation, Gandhi settled in the Transvaal in order to support Indian rights. He chose Johannesburg, the town with the largest Indian population in the province,* as his new base.

Large-scale Indian passive resistance was launched on 11 September 1906 at an angry mass meeting in Johannesburg's old Empire Theatre. At least 3 000 Indians from all over the Transvaal protested against the Asiatic Law Amendment Ordinance, a measure requiring 'Asiatics' to register their fingerprints and carry registration certificates. Gandhi denounced the Ordinance as an insult to the entire Indian community in South Africa. Standing with hands raised, all present took a solemn oath, with God as witness, to resist the Ordinance if it became law.

The first priority of the Indian resistance was to block the Asiatic Law Amendment Ordinance which had to receive royal assent before it could become law. Together with Haji Ojer Ally, the first president of the Hamidia Islamic Society, Gandhi travelled to Britain to lobby against the Ordinance. Welcome news that His Majesty Edward VII had declined to support it reached Gandhi and Ally on their return journey in December 1906.

Within days, though, the Transvaal was granted responsible government and royal assent was no longer needed for the province to pass its bills. The new parliament promptly confirmed the hated Ordinance as one of its first bills in March 1907 and soon afterwards the bill became law as the Transvaal Asiatic Registration Act. Another piece of discriminatory legislation – the Transvaal Immigration Restriction Act of 1907 – restricted the entry of Indians into the Transvaal. Passive resistance galvanised around this pair of anti-Indian laws, and was later broadened to include other issues as well.

That the resistance would be free from violence was clear from the outset. But in those early days Gandhi did not explain exactly what methods and techniques would be used and was, himself, probably unclear about them. The principles and methods would evolve through struggle in the ensuing months and years.

The movement unfolded in a dramatic series of events with the Transvaal, and especially Johannesburg, being the main centre of resistance from 1906 to 1912. This was, Gandhi realised, a truly momentous struggle:

---

* Accurate estimates of the size of the Indian population in the Transvaal during these early days are few and far between. About 1 500 Indians lived in Johannesburg in 1897 but by the end of the Anglo-Boer War in 1902 there were no more than 2 000 Indians in the whole Transvaal. By 1904 that number had risen to 10 000, and according to Gandhi, in 1909 there were 13 000.

In my opinion this struggle of the Indians in the Transvaal is the greatest of modern times, inasmuch as it has been idealised both as to the goal as also to the methods adopted to reach the goal. I am not aware of a struggle in which the participants are not to derive any personal advantage at the end of it and in which 50 percent of the persons affected have undergone great suffering and trial for the sake of a principle.

Letter to Leo Tolstoy, 10 November 1909

Gandhi chose the term Satyagraha to describe his struggle, stressing that it was different from what people generally meant in English by the phrase 'passive resistance'. Loosely translated as 'truth force', Satyagraha is essentially a philosophy of non-violent non-cooperation which calls for self-sacrifice and willingness to undergo suffering without resorting to violence no matter what the provocation.

Of the adoption of the name which has become synonymous with his own, Gandhi wrote:

As the struggle advanced, the phrase 'passive resistance' gave rise to confusion and it appeared shameful to permit this great struggle to be known only by an English name. A small prize was therefore announced in 'Indian Opinion' to be awarded to the reader who invented the best designation for our struggle. … Shri Maganlal Gandhi was one of the competitors and he suggested the word sadragraha, meaning 'firmness in a good cause'. I liked the word but it did not fully represent the whole idea I wished it to connote. I therefore corrected it to satyagraha. Truth (satya) implies love, and firmness (agraha) engenders and therefore serves as a synonym for force. I thus began to call the Indian movement satyagraha, that is to say, the Force which is born of Truth and Love or non-violence, and gave up the use of the phrase 'passive resistance' in connection with it.

Satyagraha spread to Natal in 1913 when Indian coal miners and indentured labourers went on strike. Thousands were arrested in this climactic campaign. In July 1914 Gandhi reached a settlement with the government, ending eight years of struggle, but he left many issues for his lieutenants to address when he went to bring Satyagraha to India.

His international reputation, acquired during his time in South Africa, ensured Gandhi entrée into the top ranks of the nationalist leadership in India. The moral doctrines and political techniques he carried from Africa needed only to be refined. Armed with these, he became an inspired leader in his homeland.

Gandhi's impact was also felt within South Africa's black liberation movement. The founders of the African National Congress (ANC) in 1912 witnessed and were deeply influenced by Satyagraha. Gandhi s political technique, and even elements of his philosophy, became an enduring legacy for the continuing struggle against racial discrimination in South Africa.

The first mass anti-apartheid campaign, the Defiance Campaign organised by the ANC and the South African Indian Congress in 1952, remained close to the pattern of passive resistance set by Gandhi. Africans disobeyed pass laws and curfew regulations; Indian and African volunteers walked up to 'whites only' counters in post offices and other public buildings; and whites and Indians entered African townships illegally. More than 8 000 volunteers arrested for defying apartheid laws refused to pay fines, serving prison sentences instead.

For the first half century of its existence, the African National Congress remained implacably opposed to violence but, by the early 1960s, with the organisation banned and forced underground, its leadership concluded that only through armed struggle could the ANC achieve its goal of liberation.

While direct Gandhian influence on the anti-apartheid struggle waned, non-violence was ultimately vindicated and became a decisive force in the defeat of apartheid. Protests led by the United Democratic Front in the 1980s signalled a major revival of non-violent struggle.

Armed struggle did not seriously threaten the military might of the apartheid state. Non-violent mass action, combined with international economic pressure, proved more telling, ultimately forcing the oppressor to the negotiation table. Change through negotiation, using mass action to force concessions from the oppressor, is an essential part of the Gandhian method. During his South African struggle Gandhi repeatedly engaged in talks with Jan Smuts, his main political opponent. More recently Nelson Mandela and the African National Congress engaged the white government of F W de Klerk in negotiations which led to the end of apartheid.

The force of Gandhi's example is undoubted. Some, like the Reverend Martin Luther King in the United States, accepted Satyagraha as the only morally sound method open to oppressed people in their struggle for freedom. Many others adopted passive resistance methods for reasons that were largely tactical or practical. Gandhi himself was a skilled tactician as well as a great moralist. These qualities, together with his idiosyncratic style, produced a champion of non-violence who is unmatched in modern times.

This book explores aspects of the cultural, social and political context in which his unique philosophy was worked out.

Founded as a mining camp in 1886, Johannesburg became the fastest growing urban settlement in the world. Gandhi was struck by the town's prodigious energy and coarse materialism:

Johannesburg is full of bustle … It would be no exaggeration to say that the citizens of Johannesburg do not walk but seem as if they run. No one has the leisure to look at anyone else, and everyone is apparently engrossed in thinking how to amass the maximum wealth in the minimum of time!

Amidst this scramble for wealth, people of colour (including Indians) were often trampled underfoot. All Indians came to be called Coolies - originally meaning Indian labourers - in an insulting and derogatory sense. As Gandhi stated in a radio interview recorded towards the end of his life for the British Broadcasting Corporation:

I was, with my countrymen, in a hopeless minority, not only a hopeless minority but a despised minority. If the Europeans of South Africa will forgive me for saying so, we were all Coolies. I was an insignificant Coolie lawyer. At that time we had no Coolie doctors. We had no Coolie lawyers. I was the first in the field. Nevertheless, [I was] a Coolie.

Slum conditions prevailed in the locations for Indians, Coloureds and Africans. These areas, situated near the margins of the white town, were usually on or near swampy or poorly drained land. Gandhi himself never lived in an Indian location, but occupied a succession of homes in white areas.

He was constantly on the move, ranging far and wide within the Johannesburg area. Not only did he change houses often, he also walked tirelessly.

During his student days in London Gandhi had walked an average of 16 kilometres a day and during his years in Johannesburg, the man who would in time lead marches against the British Empire across vast distances in India was confirmed as a lifelong walker.

Initially, because Johannesburg's horse drawn trams were reserved for whites (then known as 'Europeans') only, Gandhi felt obliged to walk between home and office. When electric trams began running in February 1906 they, too, were generally reserved 'For Europeans'. While living in Troyeville he walked the six kilometres to and from his office. During his stay in Bellevue-East, he walked still further between home and office, both ways. Later, while living in the far-flung suburb of Orchards with his friend Hermann Kallenbach, both men walked ten kilometres to their offices in town, even though Kallenbach could ride the trams. But this pales in comparison to the thirty-five kilometre journey made by Gandhi and his followers from their settlement at Tolstoy Farm. Gandhi explains the routine:

> *Anyone who wished to go to Johannesburg went there on foot once or twice a week and returned the same day. … The general practice was that the sojourner would rise at two o'clock and start at half past two. He would reach Johannesburg in six to seven hours. The record for the minimum time taken on the journey was four hours and eighteen minutes.*

Tolstoy Farm and the other places and buildings described here are landmarks of Gandhi's personal and political growth. The sites span huge social divides – from the slums and shanties of Coolie Location to comfortable white suburbs across town. Considered as a whole, these sites and the events surrounding them are an essential part of the Gandhi experience.

CITY OF GOLD

FOUNDED AS a gold-rush town in 1886, Johannesburg probably grew faster than any other city in the world. By the early 1890s Johannesburg was larger than Cape Town, which was then 250 years old.

But the birthmarks of Johannesburg's rough early days were slow to fade. For Albert West, one of Gandhi's closest friends, golden Johannesburg left much to be desired:

> *I was not favourably impressed with Johannesburg, which, just after the Boer War [1899-1902], was no better than a mining camp, many of the buildings being of wood and iron, including the Municipal Offices. The Market Square was a huge sandy area large enough for a span of sixteen oxen to swing around with its long wagon load of farm produce. Even the main streets were rough tracks which would often become impassable during a dust storm.*

Johannesburg was known as the Golden City, and the glowing tales of its wealth led one to believe that its streets were paved with gold. I learnt when I visited a gold mine that gold was never found in nuggets in the reef mines but in small particles contained in rocks which, by a milling process, came out in grains which were melted into gold bars. Some of this gold ore contained so little gold that it did not pay to process it. So this was used as a road-making material and made the streets of gold.

From *In the Early Days With Gandhi* by Albert West

GANDHI

IN

TOWN

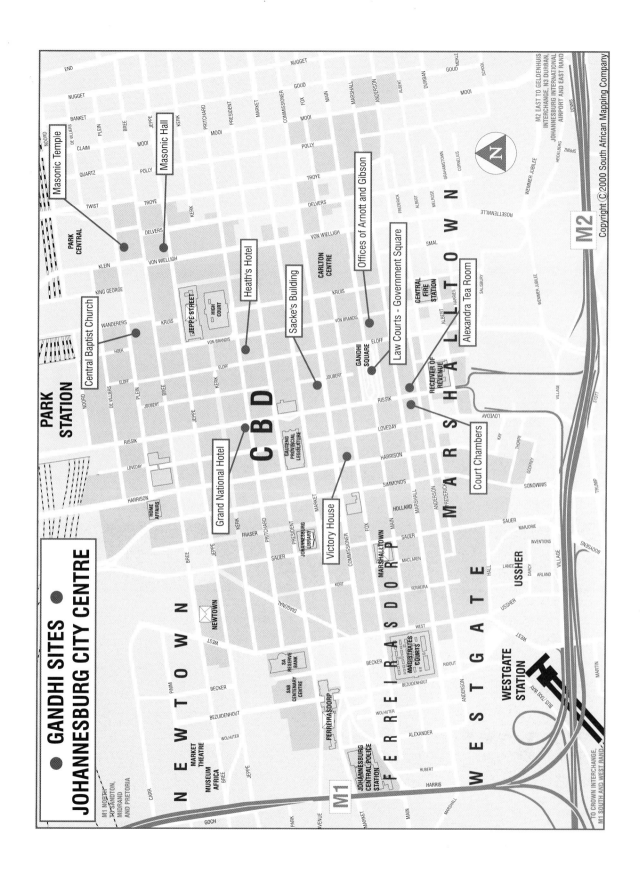

GANDHI SITES
JOHANNESBURG CITY CENTRE

PARK STATION

CBD

NEWTOWN

MARSHALLTOWN

FERREIRASDORP

WESTGATE

Masonic Temple
Masonic Hall
Central Baptist Church
Heath's Hotel
Sacke's Building
Offices of Arnott and Gibson
Law Courts - Government Square
Alexandra Tea Room
Court Chambers
Grand National Hotel
Victory House

HIGH COURT
JEPPE STREET
CARLTON CENTRE
GANDHI SQUARE
CENTRAL FIRE STATION
RECEIVER OF REVENUE
GAUTENG PROVINCIAL LEGISLATURE
JOHANNESBURG LIBRARY
HOME AFFAIRS
MARKET THEATRE
MUSEUM AFRICA
SA RESERVE BANK
SAB CENTENARY CENTRE
MAGISTRATES COURTS
JOHANNESBURG CENTRAL POLICE STATION
WESTGATE STATION

PARK CENTRAL

M1
M2

M1 NORTH
TO SANDTON,
MIDRAND
AND PRETORIA

M2 EAST TO GELDENHUIS
INTERCHANGE, N3 DURBAN,
JOHANNESBURG INTERNATIONAL
AIRPORT AND EAST RAND

TO CROWN INTERCHANGE,
M1 SOUTH AND WEST RAND

Copyright © 2000 South African Mapping Company

GRAND NATIONAL HOTEL
Corner of Rissik and Pritchard Streets. Edgars City now covers this area.

AS a twenty-three year old, newly-arrived in South Africa, Gandhi had a short but revealing stopover in Johannesburg. In his biography he recalls how he was refused accommodation at the Grand National Hotel on about 5 June 1893.

I saw the Manager and asked for a room. He eyed me for a moment, and politely saying 'I am very sorry, we are full up', bade me good-bye.[1]

Gandhi found a host in Abdul Gani, an Indian merchant who had a hearty laugh over the newcomer's experience at the hotel. The account from the autobiography continues:

'How ever did you expect to be admitted to a hotel?' he said. 'Why not?' I asked. 'You will come to know after you have stayed here a few days,' said he. Only we can live in a land like this, because, for making money, we do not mind pocketing insults, and here we are.' With this he narrated for me the story of the hardships of Indians in South Africa.

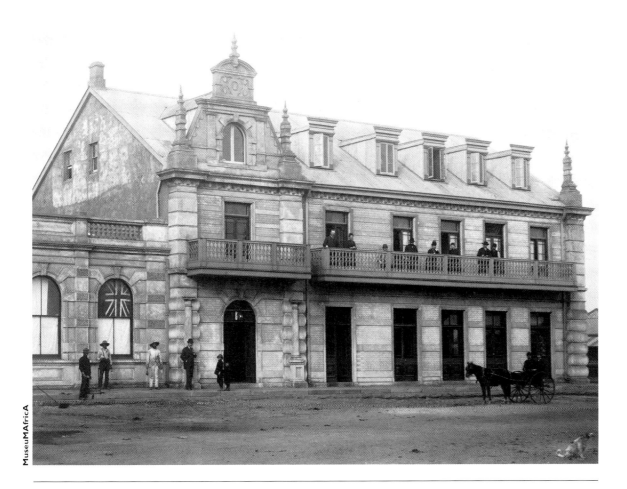

MuseuMAfricA

No room? Newly arrived from India, Gandhi was turned away from the Grand National Hotel

9

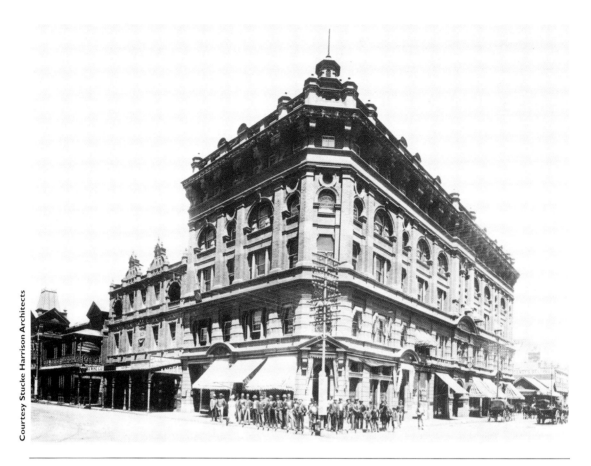

Courtesy Stucke Harrison Architects

Victory House, where Johannesburg's first lift had crowds gaping for weeks

VICTORY HOUSE (ALSO KNOWN AS PERMANENT BUILDINGS)

34 Harrison Street, at the corner of Commissioner Street.

THE LIFT at Permanent Buildings (now Victory House) was installed in 1898 and is believed to have been the first in Johannesburg. Other lifts had been tried in the new building, but this was the only one to give complete satisfaction. Not only a technological marvel, complete with a safety apparatus, it also boasted a polished oak cage.[2]

Historian Eric Rosenthal, whose father had his offices at Permanent Buildings, has written of his

father's first personal encounter with Gandhi on the day the caretaker-cum-lift operator in the building, an ex-policeman named Hallet, refused to convey him in the lift.[3]

Gandhi had probably gone to the building for an appointment with Mrs Carrie Chapman Catt, a prominent American suffragette. While visiting Johannesburg in 1911 Mrs Catt sent Gandhi an invitation to call at her hotel. She records their on-off meeting in her diary:

At the hour named a pretty, intelligent young Russian Jewess called and explained that she was Mr Gandhi's secretary and that no Indian was permitted to enter a hotel to call upon a guest. A prominent lawyer to whom I told the tale offered the use of his office for the purpose of an interview, so again I wrote, stating the time and place when I would be glad to receive him. Again the pretty little Jewess came to the lawyer's office to say that Mr. Gandhi had come but the elevator operator refused to take him up and **he would not so far demean himself as to walk when the European was carried.** *This challenged my curiosity and I told the young girl to tell him to go back to his office and that I would call upon him. Directly Miss Cameron and I, escorted by the secretary, were on our way. She took us into quarters apparently occupied exclusively by Indians … We found the man seated behind an American desk – a small very black man with his head wrapped in a very white turban* [my emphasis].[4]

⁕

GANDHI had for many years been keen to promote vegetarianism. He often dined at Johannesburg's vegetarian restaurants, and supported them financially. Adolf Ziegler, a German health enthusiast who practised Kuhne's hydropathic treatment, owned the town's first vegetarian establishment. Its second, the Alexandra Tea Room, was started by the artist Miss A M Bissicks. The existence of both these eateries was colourful but all too brief.

Albert West described an encounter with Gandhi at Ziegler's establishment:

I first met Gandhi in a vegetarian restaurant in Johannesburg in 1903. Around a large table sat a mixed company of men comprising a stockbroker from the United States who operated on the Exchange in gold and diamond shares, an accountant from Natal, a machinery agent, a young Jewish member of the Theosophical Society, a working tailor from Russia, Gandhi the lawyer, and me a printer. Everybody in Johannesburg talked about the share market, but these men were food reformers interested in vegetarian diet, Kuhne baths, earth poultices, fasting, etc.[5]

Despite Gandhi's patronage, the business he brought by taking friends there, and the money he donated, Ziegler's restaurant was always in financial difficulties and it came as no surprise when it was forced to close.[6]

THE ALEXANDRA TEA ROOM[7]
First floor Livingstone Buildings, 18 Rissik Street. Annuity House now stands on this site.

MISS BISSICKS opened the Alexandra at Livingstone Buildings, just a stone's throw from Gandhi's offices, in October 1904. Years later Gandhi would ruefully recall that not only was Miss Bissicks enterprising, she was also extravagant and ignorant of accounts[8]. But to begin with Gandhi had no inkling that she was less than financially responsible.

After starting her tea room in a small way, Miss Bissicks decided to extend her facilities on a grand scale. Money was needed for large rooms and she told Gandhi of her plans.

Gandhi was able to help. Because of his reputation for honesty, some of his clients entrusted him with large amounts of money as deposits. One such client, named Badri, was a former indentured labourer who put all his trust in Gandhi. On the strength of Gandhi's recommendation, Badri agreed to loan £1 000 for the expansion of the Alexandra.

The restaurant failed and Badri's money was lost. A worried Gandhi, guilty of an error of

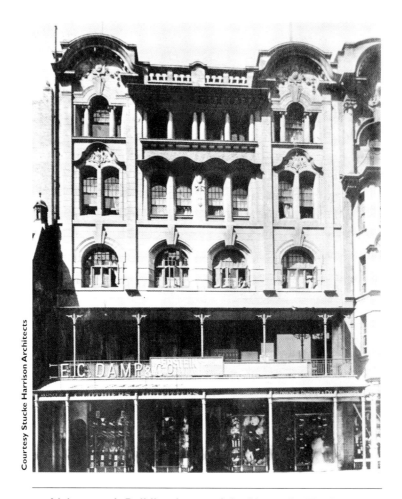

Livingstone's Building, home of the Alexandra Tea Room

judgement, undertook to repay his unfortunate client, and the high income brought in by his law practice enabled him to restore Badri's money within a year.

The experience was a chastening one for Gandhi (though it failed to dampen his commitment to vegetarianism) and he began to take more seriously the rebukes of his friends who had often advised him to exercise more care in financial matters. 'The error became for me a beaconlight of warning,' Gandhi later reflected[9]. As for Badri, he went on to play a prominent part in Satyagraha and suffered imprisonment for the cause.

COURT CHAMBERS
15 Rissik Street, between Anderson and Marshall Streets.

COURT CHAMBERS, which derived its name from the law courts located nearby in Government Square, was probably opposite the Alexandra Tea Room on a site that currently serves as a car park. With its close proximity to the courts, the building was ideally positioned for lawyers' offices. Gandhi continued to keep offices at Court Chambers until at least 1910.

He had found rooms there with assistance from

Lewis Ritch, his articled clerk, and the estate agent, C H Kew, and as early as 1904 he appeared among the attorneys listed in *Donaldson and Hill's Transvaal and Rhodesia directory*: Gandhi, M K, 25 and 26 Court Chambers. Later he moved to numbers 21 and 24[10]. The *United Transvaal Directory for* 1908 records that Gandhi, M K, attorney, was at 21 to 24 Court Chambers, at the corner of Rissik and Anderson Streets.

On 10 May 1903 Gandhi wrote from his newly acquired offices to Gopal K Gokhale, the Indian statesman, mentioning that he had settled in Johannesburg under great difficulties.

His first home, from 1903 to 1904, was in a rented room behind the offices at the southern end of Rissik Street, between Anderson and Marshall Streets. He left these single quarters late in 1904[11], moving to a family home in Troyeville with his wife and children. Henry Polak, an attorney in Gandhi's firm, recalled that:

> *At the time of our first meeting, as his family was still in India, he was living in a modest room behind his chambers in Rissik Street. A little later, and when he had settled down with the family as a small householder, he offered me its use, which helped to bring me into closer contact with him[12].*

Gandhi's first biographer, the Rev Joseph Doke, described the unpretentious interior of Gandhi's workplace:

> *The office, at the corner of Rissik and Anderson Streets, I found to be like other*
>
> *offices. It was intended for work and not for show. The windows and door were adorned with the name of the occupant with the denomination of Attorney attached to it. The first room was given up to a lady-typist; the second, into which I was ushered, was the SANCTUM SANCTORUM. It was meagrely furnished and dusty. A few pictures were scattered along the walls. They were chiefly photographs of no great merit. The Indian Stretcher-bearer Corps was in evidence – photographs of Mrs Besant, Sir William Wilson Hunter, and Justice Ranade – several separate Indian portraits – and a beautiful picture of Jesus Christ. Some indifferent chairs, and shelves filled with law books completed the inventory.[13]*

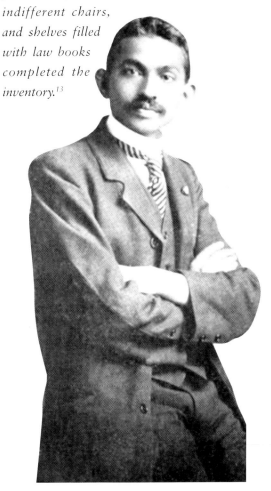

Successful lawyer. Gandhi ran a flourishing law firm, but political preoccupations eventually brought his legal work to a standstill

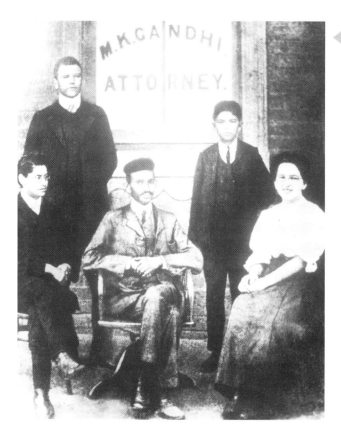

Gandhi with Henry Polak and his secretary
Sonja Schlesin outside his law office

The Court Chambers offices were also the
headquarters of the Satyagraha Association.
Here, photographed in front of Court
Chambers in 1908 is Gandhi (third from left)
with Indian and Chinese passive resistance
leaders.

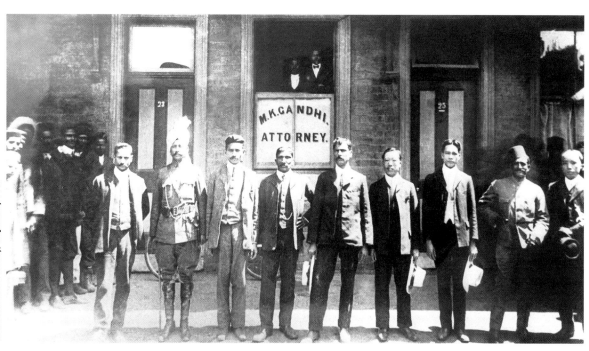

Transvaal Leader Weekly, 11 January 1908

As Johannesburg's only Indian attorney, as well as one of the most prominent Indians in the country, Gandhi's services were in great demand. He held retainers from leading Indian traders, but his office also served poorer sections of the community. A series of anti-Indian laws brought him many clients. He built a lucrative practice which, at its peak, brought him £5 000 a year, but as passive resistance intensified, he was increasingly drawn into the political arena, to the detriment of the practice.

Gandhi's offices became the headquarters of the Transvaal British Indian Association and the centre of anti-government agitation. His income supported political work, communal settlements at Phoenix and Tolstoy Farm, and the newspaper *Indian Opinion* which he founded in 1903. *Indian Opinion* became the movement's main propaganda instrument but it ran at a loss from its inception and ensuring the newspaper's survival during its first few years exhausted almost all Gandhi's savings[14].

Lewis Ritch and Henry Polak gradually took over the day-to-day running of the firm, and Ritch eventually bought it outright in 1911.

LAW COURTS
Government Buildings, Government Square (now Gandhi Square).

THE WITWATERSRAND High Court and Magistrates Courts were located in Government Square, which was bounded by Rissik, Eloff, Fox and Marshall Streets. The ground originally belonged to Goldfields Club, which built an impressive clubhouse in the middle of this area. Before the interior was completed the government bought the building and the land surrounding it. The building was converted into a courthouse in about 1893. It was then that the area was named Government Square[15].

The old High Court went out of use in 1911, when the present Supreme Court Building in Pritchard Street arose at Von Brandis Square.

The old law courts were demolished in 1948, to make way for Johannesburg's main bus terminus. The City Council renamed the area Van der Byl Square the following year[16] in honour of the first chairman of the parastatal Electricity Supply Commission (Escom), Dr Hendrik Johannes Van der Byl. Towering over the square, at the corner of Rissik and Main Streets, was the twenty-one storey Escom House. But the area's physical link with Dr Van der Byl was broken when Escom House was imploded in 1983.

Van der Byl Square became increasingly unsafe and squalid during the 1990s, adding to the general air of deterioration in the central town area. But by the close of the decade it had become the centrepiece of efforts to revive the central business district and restore confidence in the city centre.

The square was upgraded by the Central Johannesburg Partnership, a private sector organisation dedicated to urban renewal, and the revamped square is managed as an urban improvement district financed by a self-imposed levy borne by the surrounding property owners. The special levy pays for improving public services like security and cleaning beyond that provided by the municipality. About 40 percent of the square is used as a bus terminus, while the rest has been paved and landscaped.

The area was renamed in 1999 to coincide with the upgrading and, following a proposal from MuseuMAfricA, has been renamed Gandhi Square. Panels mounted on the square supply information about the Indian leader's connection with the area.

Many of those for whom Gandhi appeared in court were Satyagrahis charged with failing to register for passes, picketing, and other political offences. In their defence Gandhi not only presented legal arguments, but also drew the court's attention to moral and ethical considerations. The law, he argued, violated the conscience of the accused.

Gandhi also appeared in a Johannesburg court as a defendant in two political trials. The first was held at Johannesburg's B Criminal Court on 28 December 1907. Having refused to register under the Transvaal Asiatic Registration Act, Gandhi and twenty-six of his comrades were summoned to appear before the magistrate, Mr H H Jordan. The court ordered Gandhi to leave the Transvaal within forty-eight hours.

He did not do so and on 10 January 1908 he was arrested and again brought before Mr Jordan. Inside the crowded courtroom were hundreds of Indians as well as fellow legal practitioners. In his book, *Satyagraha in South Africa*, Gandhi recalls:

I had some slight feeling of awkwardness due to the fact that I was standing as an accused in the very Court where I had often appeared as counsel. But I well remember that I considered the former role as far more honourable than the latter, and did not feel the slightest hesitation in entering the prisoner's box.[17]

Gandhi asked for the maximum penalty - six months imprisonment with hard labour and a fine of £500. Mr Jordan did not oblige, but sentenced him to two months in jail (his first term of imprisonment). After sentence was passed, Gandhi was held for a few minutes in the prisoners' yard attached to the court. Then, in order to evade the huge crowd gathered outside, he was stealthily taken to a covered van, and quickly driven to the Fort Prison.

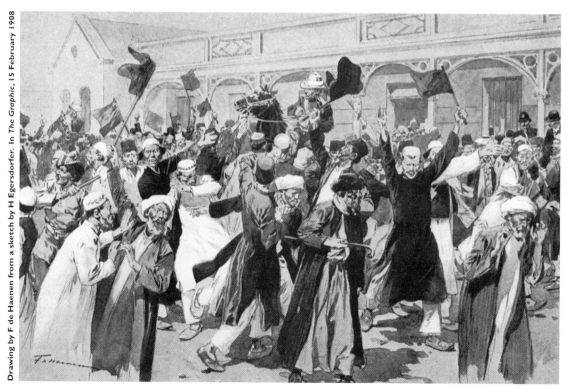

Drawing by F de Haenen from a sketch by H Egersdorfer. In *The Graphic*, 15 February 1908

OFFICES OF
ARNOTT AND GIBSON

29 Von Brandis Street. This site, at the south-west corner of Von Brandis and Main Streets is now occupied by Byron House.

ON 10 FEBRUARY 1908 Gandhi nearly lost his life in the street outside Arnott and Gibson's law offices when he was assaulted by a militant group who believed he had betrayed them.

The event which precipitated the attack was the promulgation of the Asiatic Registration Act (Transvaal Act 2 of 1907) which made it compulsory for Asians to carry passes and to register for them by giving fingerprints. Gandhi campaigned against the Act and led a successful boycott of the registration process in the early phase of his passive resistance campaign. But by 30 January 1908, he had agreed to support voluntary registration, as part of a compromise with General Smuts, then Transvaal Colonial Secretary. The government, for its part, undertook (according to Gandhi's understanding) to abolish compulsory registration and repeal the Act once the majority of Indians had registered voluntarily. Smuts may have understood the settlement differently.[18]

Though many Indians still opposed registration under any circumstances, Gandhi decided that, to carry out his part of the compromise, he would set an example by being the first Indian to register voluntarily.

Gandhi was accompanied to the Registration Office by Essop Mia, Chairman of the British Indian Association, and C K Thambi Naidoo, the great Tamil leader and, effectively, Gandhi's deputy in Johannesburg. As they walked from Gandhi's office to the Registration Office in Von Brandis Square to give their fingerprints, the three were attacked by militant Pathans – led by Mir Alam Khan – who viewed the compromise of January 1908 as a betrayal.

Gandhi described the assault in the *Indian Opinion* of 22 February 1908:

I do not remember the manner of the assault, but people say that I fell down unconscious with the first blow which was delivered with a stick. Then my assailants struck me with an iron pipe and a stick, and they also kicked me. Thinking me dead, they stopped.

Some of the blows were warded off by Gandhi's companions, who were themselves badly beaten. Gandhi was carried, semi-conscious, into Gibson's office. Hundreds of Indians soon gathered outside, and the entrance was guarded by policemen.

Knowing of Gandhi's intention to register, Baptist Minister Joseph Doke had gone to the Registration Office that morning, borne by a vague sense of portent. 'I remember particularly that morning being led to pray as I went through the streets, especially that I might be guided completely to do God's word, but I little thought what the answer would be,' Doke was to reflect later

At that point, Doke had met Gandhi only briefly, but they already shared a bond of sympathy. Doke was a courageous and dedicated social reformer who was quick to identify with the Indian struggle. As a former passive resister himself, Doke could hardly fail to be impressed by Gandhi's efforts. While in Britain Doke had supported the passive resistance waged by Nonconformist churches against the Education Act of 1902.

News of the attack on Gandhi and his companions reached Doke who was, at the time,

◄ A demonstration outside the courts after Gandhi and five others were sentenced in January 1908. Mounted police dispersed the crowd

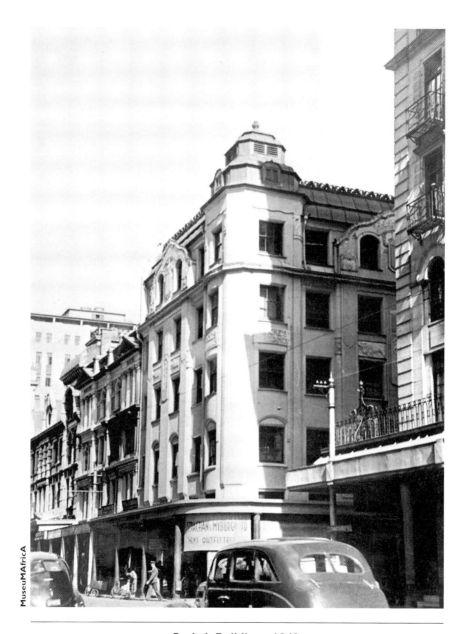

Sacke's Building, c1940

talking to Henry Polak at the Registration Office. Together they rushed to find Gandhi, and pushed their way into Gibson's Office. Doke recorded the scene in his diary:

I found Mr Gandhi lying on the floor looking half dead, while the doctor was cleaning the wounds on his face and lips. Mr Thambi Naidoo, with a severe scalp wound and blood all over his collar and coat, was describing the assault to some policemen. Mr Isop [sic] Mia, with a gash across his head, was also there. When the doctor had finished with Mr Gandhi, I went over and he recognised me. Then the question was mooted; where should he be taken?

He was badly knocked about, his face cut open right through the lip, an ugly swelling over the eye, and his side so bruised that he could hardly move; there might be complications. Some said: Take him to the Hospital. I had hardly time to think, but it seemed as though God had led me there for a purpose and possibly this purpose. So I said: If he would like to come home with me, we shall be glad to have him[19].

On being asked where he wanted to go, Gandhi seemed indifferent, and used what little strength he had to insist that no action be taken to punish his attackers. Still barely conscious, he was conveyed in a carriage to the manse of the Rev Doke to recuperate.

SACKE'S BUILDINGS
23/25/27 Joubert Street (corner of Joubert and Commissioner Streets).

SACKE'S BUILDINGS housed the offices of Hermann Kallenbach, Gandhi's friend and supporter. Kallenbach, a prosperous German-Jewish architect, designed and built Sacke's Buildings in 1903-4. One of Kallenbach's major projects, commissioned by his uncles Henri and Simon Sacke, the design reflected the Swiss-German architecture of the time.[20] The building was distinctively white with almost square windows. Kallenbach and Reynolds occupied the fourth floor[21].

Given Gandhi's close relationship with Kallenbach, it is probable that he occasionally called on Kallenbach at his office, particularly as it was only two minutes' walk from Gandhi's office.

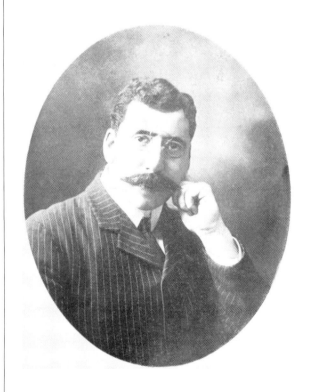

Hermann Kallenbach ▶

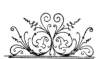
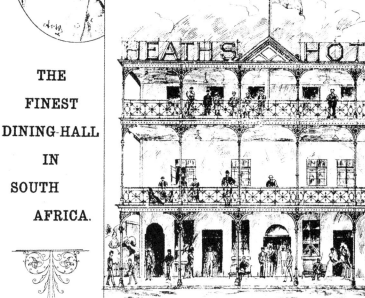

HEATH'S HOTEL

78 Pritchard Street. The Eloff Street Branch of OK Bazaars, which occupies the whole block, now covers this site.

WILLIAM HEATH established his luxurious and exclusive three-storey hotel in the early 1890s. The dining room on the ground floor was particularly grand: a lofty, elegantly arranged banqueting hall capable of accommodating a large number of guests.

Lewis Ritch recounts how Gandhi was admitted to the hotel, but denied access to this dining room:

Exactly at what stage in our association it was I can't recall, but Gandhiji required (it must have been on the occasion of one of his visits to Johannesburg) hotel accommodation for a short period. Heath's was the leading hotel at the time, so I interviewed Heath personally in the matter. Heath was a kindly soul, but also a licensed hotel-keeper whose patrons were rather superior people and more than likely to resent the presence of Indians as fellow-guests. Poor Heath was torn between a desire to accommodate and his dread of repercussions. Eventually we arrived at a compromise. If Mr Gandhi would take his meals in a lobby instead of in the public dining room, the difficulty might be overcome. With characteristic consideration for his host's dilemma Gandhiji agreed; he and I dined together and the superior people were spared the indignity of our company.[22]

Advertisement for Heath's Hotel

MASONIC HALL

95 Jeppe Street. The Medical Centre building occupies this site, which is now 202 Jeppe Street.[23]

GANDHI gave a lecture on Hinduism at the Masonic Hall on 18 August 1903 to the Johannesburg Lodge of the Theosophical Society. Although he himself was not a theosophist, he had many friends in the Society of which a branch had been established in Johannesburg in 1899. Among the small group of theosophists Gandhi met after he settled in the town were Miss Bissicks; Lewis Ritch; Herbert Kitchin, an engineer who settled in Phoenix; Lewis Playford, the Chief Magistrate of Johannesburg; and William Wybergh, the Commissioner of Mines.

Theosophy drew heavily on eastern religious concepts – Buddhism, Islamic Sufism, Taoism, and especially Hinduism. The Theosophical Society founded in New York by the religious mystic Helena Blavatsky and others in 1875 became the first modern western cult with a strong Hindu influence.

The theosophists looked to Gandhi as an expert on Hinduism, a role for which he felt ill-equipped:

Theosophical literature is replete with Hindu influence, and so these friends expected that I should be helpful to them. I explained that my Sanskrit study was not much to speak of, that I had not read the Hindu scriptures in the original, and that even my acquaintance with the translations was of the slightest. But being believers in samskara (tendencies caused by previous births) and punarjanma (rebirth), they assumed that I should be able to render at least some help.[24]

Gandhi read a great deal of Hindu religious philosophy with the theosophists, and was persuaded to lecture to their society on several occasions. In his talk of 18 August 1903 he recalled being asked to expound the *Bhagavad Gita* to a theosophical group in London and realised that he needed to study it more himself before he could teach others.[25] He was grateful to the theosophists for directing his attention to his own spiritual heritage. Stimulated by them, the young Gandhi studied the *Bhagavad Gita* more deeply and memorised much of it.

On 18 February 1910, the Indian community gave a banquet at the Masonic Hall in honour of the Rev Joseph Doke. Gandhi delivered an affectionate tribute to the clergyman who had nursed him two years earlier.[26]

Gandhi was also among the speakers at a banquet for Indian statesman, G K Gokhale, held at the Hall on 31 October 1912. Gokhale arrived on a tour of the Union of South Africa at Gandhi's invitation in October 1912, and remained in South Africa until November of that year. The banquet was given by the British Indian Association and attended by 500 guests.[27]

Gandhi paid a final visit to the Masonic Hall – for his own farewell banquet – on 14 July 1914, while preparing to leave South Africa.[28] The dinner was given by the British Indian Association in honour of Gandhi, his wife Kasturba, and Kallenbach. Despite the injustices he had encountered in Johannesburg, Gandhi held the place especially dear and had formed deep personal attachments there. His speech included praise for steadfast friends and supporters, and tributes to Johannesburg's young martyrs to the passive resistance cause.

The report of his address, which was published in a special commemorative issue of *Indian Opinion* is worth quoting at length:

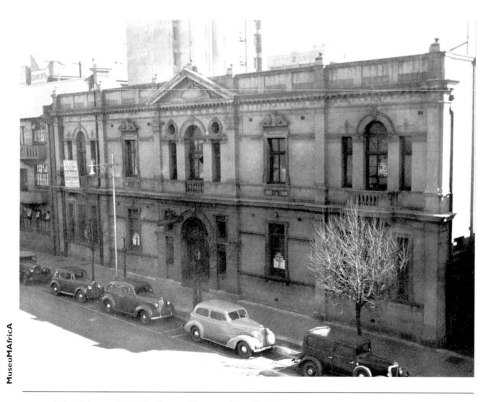

The Masonic Hall, Jeppe Street, just before it was demolished in 1940.

Johannesburg was not a new place to him. He saw many friendly faces there, many who had worked with him in many struggles in Johannesburg. He had gone through much in life. A great deal of depression and sorrow had been his lot, but he had also learnt during all those years to love Johannesburg even though it was a mining camp. It was in Johannesburg that he had found his most precious friends. It was in Johannesburg that the foundation for the great struggle of Passive Resistance was laid in the September of 1906. It was in Johannesburg that he had found a friend, a guide, and a biographer in the late Mr. Doke. It was in Johannesburg that he had found in Mrs. Doke a loving sister, who had nursed him back to life when he had been assaulted by a countryman who had misunderstood his mission and who misunderstood what he had done. It was in Johannesburg that he had found a Kallenbach, a Polak, a Miss Schlesin, and many another who had always helped him, and had always cheered him and his countrymen. Johannesburg, therefore, had the holiest associations of all the holy associations that Mrs. Gandhi and he would carry back to India, and, as he had already said on many another platform, South Africa, next to India, would be the holiest land to him and to Mrs. Gandhi and to his children, for, in spite of all the bitternesses, it had given them those life-long companions. It was in Johannesburg again that the European Committee had been formed, when Indians were going through the darkest stage in their history, presided over then, as it still was, by Mr Hosken. It was last, but not least, Johannesburg that had given Valliamma, that young girl, whose picture rose before him even as he spoke, who died in the cause of truth. Simple-minded in faith – she had not the knowledge that he had, she did not know what Passive Resistance was, she did not know what it was the community would gain, but she was simply taken up with unbounded enthusiasm for her people – she went to gaol, came out of it a wreck, and within a few days died. It was Johannesburg again that produced a Nagappen and Narayansamy, two lovely youths hardly out of their teens, who also died.[29]

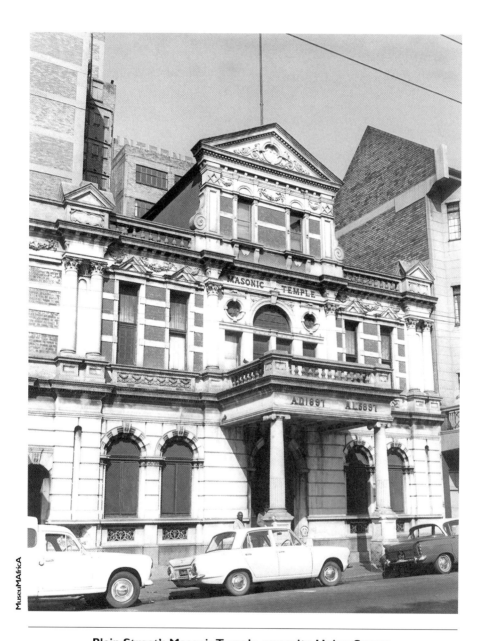

MuseuMAfricA

Plein Street's Masonic Temple, opposite Union Square

MASONIC TEMPLE
80 Plein Street. Now the site of the Union Square Building.

THE MASONIC Temple was the venue for a course of four lectures on religion delivered by Gandhi in March 1905 at the invitation of the Theosophical Society. Religious tolerance and understanding were cornerstones, Gandhi stressed, in the struggle against prejudice. *The Star* reported:

> *Mr Gandhi introduced his subject by remarking that the endeavours of the Johannesburg Lodge to promote interest in the study of different religious systems were most praiseworthy, tending, as they did, to widen peoples' sympathies, and enlarge their comprehension of the motives and beliefs underlying the actions of those who were strangers in creed and colour.*
>
> *He himself had endeavoured, during his eleven years residence in South Africa, to remove the prejudice and ignorance that existed concerning his own people[30].*

Gandhi delved deeply into Christianity and other religions including his own Hindu faith. His study of religion developed in him an acceptance of the essential validity and worth of all religions.

CENTRAL BAPTIST CHURCH
54 Plein Street (Corner of Plein and Wanderers Streets). Town Talk Furnishers now occupies the ground floor of the building at this site.

THE REV DOKE served as Minister of the Central Baptist Church from November 1907 until his death in 1913. He had left Johannesburg on a missionary journey to Central Africa in July of that year and, after falling ill on the way, he died at Umtali, Southern Rhodesia (now Mutare, Zimbabwe) on 15 August. Because of the great distance, Doke's body was not sent to Johannesburg, and the funeral took place at Umtali on 24 August 1913.[31] A memorial service was held for Doke at Johannesburg's Central Baptist Church on the same date.[32]

In a highly unusual gesture, the Church invited Gandhi to speak at the service for their late pastor – even though he was neither white nor Christian. Gandhi told the congregation that the Indian community revered Doke as one of its truest friends. His speech underlined the strong bonds forged in the sickroom:

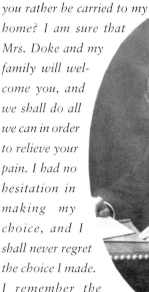
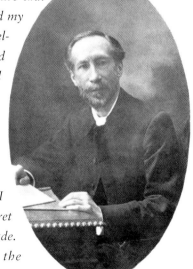

> *When I was lying in the office of a friend in a helpless condition there stood over me Mr. Doke, and his words ring in my memory today, as they were so appealing to me that afternoon. They were something like these: Would you rather go to hospital, or would you rather be carried to my home? I am sure that Mrs. Doke and my family will welcome you, and we shall do all we can in order to relieve your pain. I had no hesitation in making my choice, and I shall never regret the choice I made. I remember the*

The Rev Joseph Doke

evening when, at my request, the whole family sang to me the beautiful hymn, Lead Kindly Light. That tune will never die from my memory; it will never fade out. It is as fresh to me to-night as it was soothing on my nerves on that great evening when I saw myself surrounded by people who were no longer strangers. During the night, whether it was 12 or 1 or 2 o'clock, I could see peeping through the door, that had been purposely left open, Mr. Doke s face, just glancing in occasionally to ascertain whether I was suffering or whether I needed anything. The whole family were at my disposal in order to nourish me, in order to serve me, in order to soothe me, although I was a stranger to them and had never done a single service to them.[33]

The Church moved premises in about 1920 and the original building has long since been demolished.

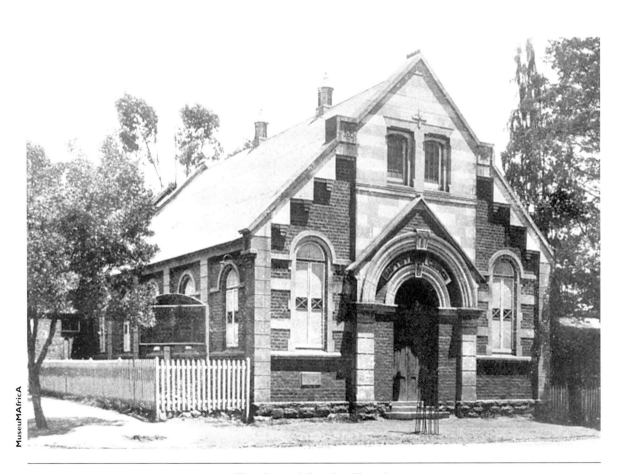

MuseuMAfricA

The Central Baptist Church

26

BRAAMFONTEIN
AND
HOSPITAL HILL

JOHANNESBURG'S old General Hospital is perched on the southern slope of the hill which separates Braamfontein and Hillbrow and has been known as Hospital Hill since 1888. Crowning the hill, and overlooking the city, is the Fort. The name Hospital Hill was also attached to places in Braamfontein and Joubert Park which are some distance from the actual hill, and which would not today be considered part of it.[34]

MANSE OF THE CENTRAL BAPTIST CHURCH

163 Smit Street, between De Beer and Melle Streets, Braamfontein. The building which now houses D J Swanepoel Butchery stands on this site.

AFTER SETTLING in Johannesburg towards the close of 1907, the Dokes took up residence at 163 Smit Street Braamfontein, in an area which was then considered part of Hospital Hill. A contemporary

Gandhi recuperates at the Doke home in Braamfontein

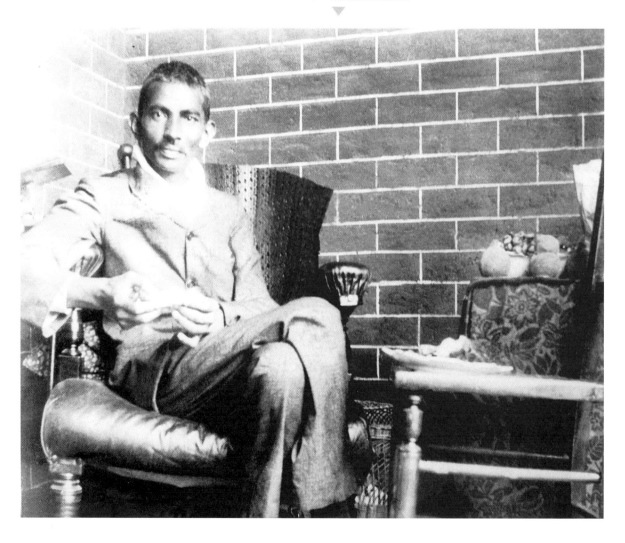

newspaper report suggests that it was to this address that Gandhi was taken after the assault of 10 February.[35] In his biography of the Rev Doke, W E Cursons notes that Gandhi was taken to the temporary manse on Hospital Hill.[36] Gandhi himself gives the name as 'Smith' Street.[37] A letter published in *The Star* of 10 January 1908 gives Doke's address as 163 Smit Street.

Another address closer to the hospital – 11 Sutherland Avenue, Hospital Hill – is given by Professor J D Hunt as the site of Doke's temporary manse.[38] Sutherland Avenue is a short cul de sac which branches off Smit but is nowhere near No 163. *The South African Baptist Handbook* indicates that the Dokes moved to Sutherland Avenue some time after Gandhi's convalescence. The Rev Doke's earliest Johannesburg address appears in the 1907-1908 edition as Hospital Hill, 163 Smit Street. His change of address is recorded in the next edition (1908-1909) as Hospital Hill, 11 Sutherland Avenue. Handbooks from 1910 to 1913 (the year of Doke's death) also give the Sutherland Avenue address.

[12] February 1908
Phoenix, Natal

Dear Mr & Mrs Doke,
Yesterday I sent a short telegraphic message thanking you for your great kindness to my father. I would now like to express more fully the thanks my mother and we all feel. When the sad news reached us my mother wished to proceed to Johannesburg at once, so great was the anxiety she felt. So it was with great relief that we heard of your kindness in taking my father to your home and giving to him the comforts of nursing and sympathy.

We can never forget your Christian and brotherly sympathy with our countrymen during the crisis and I feel sure you will receive the highest reward possible.

I remain
Yours faithfully
Harilal M. Gandhi*
per C.K. Gandhi.

14 February 1908
Phoenix, Natal

Dear & Rev. Sir,
My father writes to us that you and Mrs Doke have been treating him so well as to make him forget home in the midst of his suffering. He says that you do not give yourself any rest and that even during night you often go to his room to see if he need[s] any assistance.

My mother asks me to thank you and Mrs Doke very heartfully for all your doing for my father. She hopes that you may in the near future be able to visit the settlement at Phoenix and give us the privilege of making your personal acquaintance.

My mother is sorry that owing to her not knowing English she is unable to write to you herself.

With regards from my mother and with respects from my brothers and myself.

I remain
Yours faithfully
Harilal Gandhi

**Harilal Gandhi (1888-1948) was the eldest son of M K Gandhi

The presence of Gandhi in their home during the ten days of his recuperation earned the Dokes the disapproval of their white neighbours. The sudden influx of hundreds of Indians who came to visit Gandhi, all of whom were welcomed by the Dokes, could only have added to the neighbours' consternation.

Clement Doke, the pastor's son, witnessed these events as a schoolboy. He recalled how his home life was transformed:

I was a boy of fifteen when I first got to know Mahatma Gandhi – Mr Gandhi as he was called then – back in 1908. He was a frequent visitor at our house in Smit Street, Johannesburg, during the height of the Passive Resistance Struggle. I well remember, on coming home from school one day, being warned to enter the house quietly, for Mr Gandhi had been brought home severely injured in an assault in town. He was lying very ill in my little room off the upstairs verandah: I was proud to vacate the room to him for the days he was with us. For more than a week the house was thronged with visitors and enquirers – mostly Indian; the dining room was a mass of gifts of choice fruits sent from all parts of the Transvaal, Natal and even Lourenço Marques; and our next-door neighbours, who had been very friendly hitherto, cut us off when they knew we had taken a black man to our home. Those were great days![39]

Gandhi was sceptical of conventional Western medicine, but trusted in alternative medicine, nature cures and Indian remedies. Much to his doctor's dismay, he insisted on prescribing earth plasters for himself. Clement Doke remembered:

The healing of his wounds was slow, and he got impatient. He told my father that, if he could get a plaster of clean mud on his face, he was sure it would help. So off I was sent with spade and bucket to clean away the topsoil and get uncontaminated lower earth for the plasters. This I dug on a vacant plot of ground where now the leading Jewish Synagogue stands.

We made the mud plasters, and my mother applied them.[40]

The mud came from what would become the site of the Great Synagogue built in 1913-14 at 129 Wolmarans Street, Joubert Park. The synagogue occupies ten stands making up a complete city block bounded by Smit, Wolmarans, Claim and Quartz Streets.[41]

THE FORT PRISON COMPLEX
Hospital Hill: Bounded by Sam Hancock, Clarendon, King George, Kotze and Joubert Streets.

GANDHI was sentenced to at least four terms of imprisonment in South Africa: two in 1908, a third in 1909, and a fourth in 1913. The first of these sentences was served at the Fort in January 1908. A two-month sentence begun on 10 January ended, on General Smuts's orders, with an early release on 30 January. Gandhi was taken from prison to Smuts's offices in Pretoria for negotiations which led to a temporary settlement. Gandhi was back at the Fort on 25 October 1908 for part of his second prison term. He was transferred from Volksrust Prison to Johannesburg, where he was required to testify in a court case. A warder was specially brought from Johannesburg to escort him on the train from Volksrust. On their arrival at Johannesburg, Gandhi walked from Park Station to the Fort dressed in his prison uniform. He was taken back to Volksrust Prison on 4 November 1908.[42]

The earliest prison buildings in the Fort complex date from about 1893, when Johannesburg was only seven years old. Two cell blocks for white prisoners were erected during this period. Section Number 4, the block for black prisoners, was also built around this time. No original building plans have been found for this 'Native Gaol', but its architectural style and building materials match those of the first gaol block designed for the Transvaal government in 1892.[43]

From 1896/7 the two prison blocks for whites were surrounded by a military fortification with earth ramparts, which gave the Fort complex its name. The Fort was however used exclusively as a prison, rather than a military stronghold, from 1902 until it was closed in 1982.

The Fort's black inmates were kept segregated from their white counterparts. The prison authorities classed Indian passive resisters with the 'natives' (as Africans were then referred to). Gandhi and his compatriots were thus consigned to Section 4, the 'Native Prison'.

Section 4 was cramped, notoriously over-crowded, and small compared to the two cell blocks inside the Fort which were used for whites. Each of the 'Native' Block's thirteen cells was originally

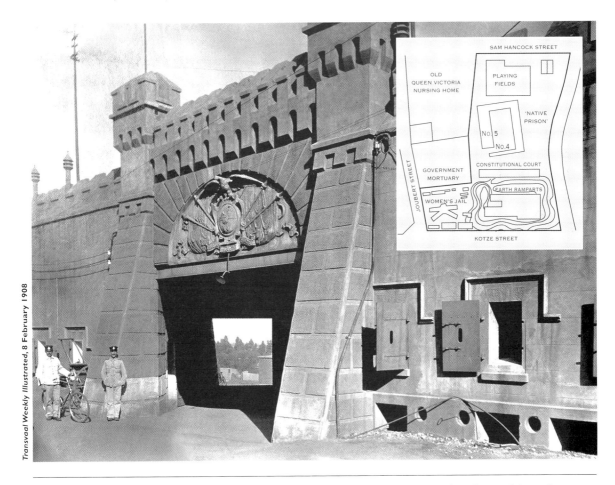

Transvaal Weekly Illustrated, 8 February 1908

The main gate of the Fort with plan of the prison complex indicating the position of Section 4, the 'Native Prison'

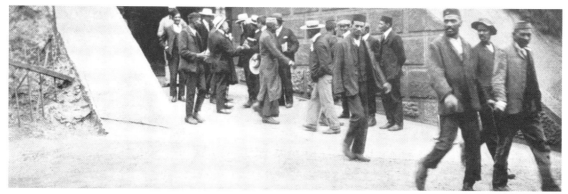

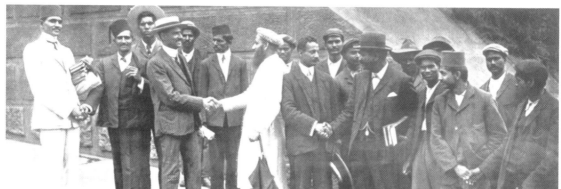

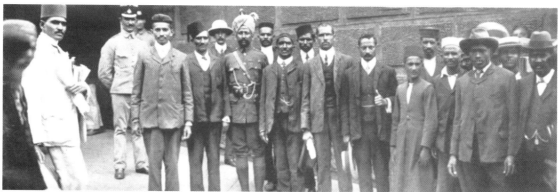

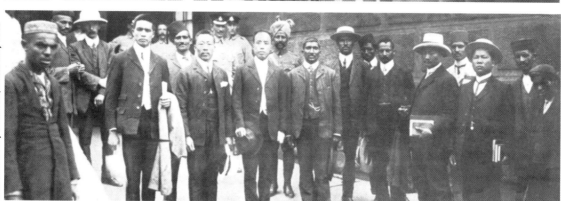

intended to house up to forty prisoners but by 1906 there were seventy-two inmates per cell.[44] When a flood of newly-arrested passive resisters arrived in January 1908, overcrowding increased still further. Gandhi takes up the story:

Our ward could accommodate 51 prisoners. The yard in front had the same capacity. When, towards the end, our number increased beyond 151, we experienced acute inconvenience. The governor ordered tents to be pitched outside, and some of us were shifted to these. During the last few days, a hundred prisoners had to sleep outside. But they were brought back every morning, with the result that the yard turned out to be too small, and it was with great difficulty that room could be found for all the prisoners ...

Anyone will admit that it was the government's fault that so many prisoners were confined in so small a place. If the space was insufficient the government ought not to have sent so many prisoners. Had the movement continued, the government would have found it impossible to accommodate any more.[45]

The old 'Native Prison' survived with few changes for ninety years until it was closed down. It is located just to the north of the site of what will be the new Constitutional Court building.

◄ **Passive resisters were released from prison following the temporary settlement of January 1908**

◄ **Receiving congratulations from friends**

◄ **Indian leaders (Gandhi is on the left)**

◄ **Chinese leaders**

PASSIVE RESISTERS' GRAVES, BRAAMFONTEIN CEMETERY
Northern side of the Cemetery, off Enoch Sontonga Avenue.

IN ONE of his last public appearances before his departure from South Africa on 18 July 1914,[46] Gandhi spoke at the unveiling of memorial stones in honour of two passive resistance martyrs, Valliamma Munusamy Moodaliar and Swami Nagappen Padayachee[47]. The ceremonial unveiling, which marked the official end of passive resistance, took place at the graves of Valliamma and Nagappen in the Hindu section of Braamfontein Cemetery on the morning of 15 July 1914. The previous evening, at his farewell banquet at the Masonic Hall, Gandhi had singled the two teenagers out for special praise.

Eighty-three years later, attention was again focused on Valliamma and Nagappen through a joint venture between the Greater Johannesburg Metropolitan Council, the Transvaal Gandhi Centenary Council, Dravidians for Peace and Justice, the Transvaal Tamil Federation, and the ANC's Lenasia Branch. Hundreds of people paid their respects on 20 April 1997 when the two graves were rededicated in the cemetery's Enoch Sontonga Memorial Park.[48]

Nagappen was about eighteen years old when he was sentenced on 21 June 1909 to £3 or ten days' imprisonment with hard labour for hawking without a permit. After spending a night at the Fort, he was made to walk to the Jukskei Road Prison Camp, a distance of 26 km. He was discharged from the camp on 30 June and died on 6 July of double pneumonia and resultant heart failure. Nagappen's body was bruised and bore weals. Fellow prisoners reported that he had been physically abused by at least one warder, and that his illness was neglected by the prison authorities – to the extent that his fellow workers had to carry him to the road works on which

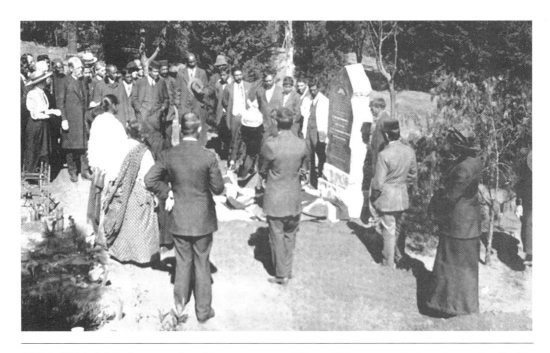

15 July 1914. A Hindu prayer is said at the grave of Swami Nagappen Padayachee, who died in 1909. Gandhi is among the assembled dignitaries

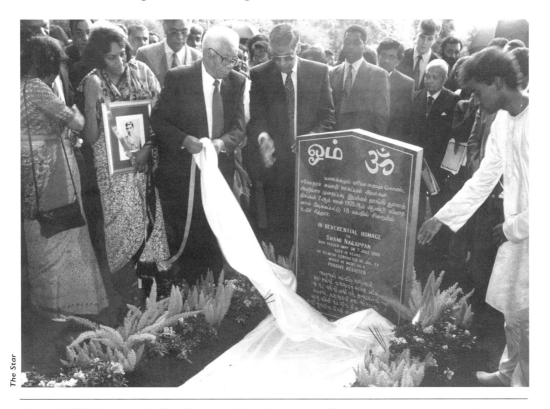

10 April 1997. Veteran ANC politician, Walter Sisulu, unveils the new tombstone for Nagappen

he was expected to carry out his sentence of hard labour. The death certificate states that he must have been ill for nine days. Despite all the evidence, the official enquiry exonerated the prison officials and rejected allegations of appalling conditions in the camp.[19]

The original English inscription on Nagappen's memorial stone read:

> *In* Loving Memory of our brother S. Nagappa Padayachy who died 6th July 1909 of pneumonia contracted in the Johannesburg-Pretoria road camp prison, to which he was taken as a passive resister.[50]

Vandals, who caused widespread damage in the cemetery, destroyed Nagappen's memorial in about 1978.[51] A new headstone and plinth slab were unveiled at the rededication ceremony in 1997.

Fortunately, the original Valliamma memorial escaped the attentions of vandals, and is still in excellent condition.[52]

It bears the inscription in English:

> *In* loving memory of our sister Valliamal Munusamy who died 22nd February 1914 aged 17 years of illness contracted in the Maritzburg gaol to which she was sent as a passive resister.[53]

The participation of women passive resisters was a key element of the Satyagraha campaign of 1913-14. Angered by a judgement in the Supreme Court in March 1913 in which a Judge Searle refused to recognise Hindu and Muslim marriages, Indian women joined the struggle for the first time. Valliamma came to symbolise the courage of these women who cast aside their traditional seclusion and braved arrest and imprisonment.

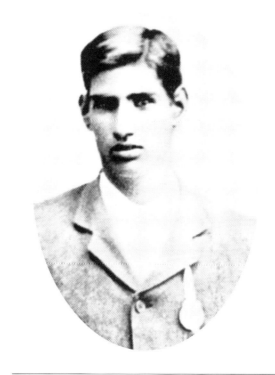

Teenage martyr, Swami Nagappen Padayachee

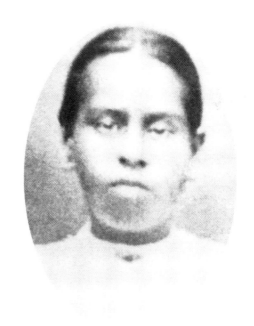

Teenage martyr, Valliamma Munusamy

The Searle judgement invalidated all Hindu and Muslim marriages, reducing married Indian women to the status of concubines, while classifying their children as illegitimate and denying them their rights of inheritance. Gandhi and the Satyagraha Association called on Indian women to join their men in protesting against these insults. In 1913, the year that also saw mass resistance of African and 'coloured' women in the Orange Free State against passes, Indian women joined the final Satyagraha campaign led by Gandhi in South Africa.

Valliamma was among hundreds of volunteers, including Johannesburg women, who suffered imprisonment. Millie Polak, in an article 'Women and the struggle', pays tribute to the women who renewed Satyagraha:

The last phase of the fight and the one through which today we rejoice in peace, was practically led in the early stages by a small band of women from Natal, who challenged prison to vindicate their right to the legal recognition of wifehood, and a similar small band of women from Johannesburg. The women from Natal, all of them wives of well-known members of the Indian community, travelled up to Volksrust and were the first of hundreds to go to gaol. The women from the Transvaal travelled down the line, taking in the mines on the way, holding meetings and calling upon the men to refuse to work and to die rather than live as slaves; and at the call of these women, thousands lay down their tools and went on strike. I think it may safely be said that, but for the early work of these brave women, the wonderful response to the call of honour and country might never have taken place.[54]

Valliamma's parents owned a fruit shop in Doornfontein, Johannesburg. At the age of sixteen (seventeen by Hindu calculation) she was among a group of women who travelled from mine to mine in Newcastle, Natal, urging indentured workers to strike. As Gandhi notes, the group was like a lighted match to dry fuel. A strike had already started when the women were arrested as vagabonds and imprisoned with hard labour. Valliamma was released from Pietermaritzburg Prison suffering from a fatal fever. She died soon afterwards, on 22 February 1914.

Both Valliamma and Nagappen were from Johannesburg's small but heroic Tamil community. As Gandhi acknowledged, the Tamils, more than any other section of the Indian community bore the brunt of the struggle.[55] The majority of women who were jailed were Tamils, as were most of the men who were repeatedly imprisoned. Tamil Satyagrahis also suffered the largest number of deaths.

Other passive resisters lie buried in unmarked graves at Braamfontein Cemetery. Foremost among them is Ahmed Mohamed Cachalia, who was laid to rest in grave number 8317 in the Muslim section. A M Cachalia became chairperson of the British Indian Association in September 1910, and led the organisation for a number of years. He was imprisoned repeatedly, and reduced to poverty as a result of his activism.

Once a rich merchant, Cachalia became insolvent when his white creditors made a concerted run on him to punish him for his role in the Indian resistance. Cachalia was a very popular figure, and highly regarded by Gandhi. In an obituary published in the *Bombay Chronicle* on 21 October 1918, Gandhi notes that among the Indians of South Africa Cachalia's prestige was unequalled. Cachalia died on 6 September 1918, aged forty-five.

Captain Jamadar Nawab Khan, a proud, turbaned figure, always immaculately turned out in his military uniform, was another prominent passive resister. The son of a major who had been killed in the second Afghan War, Nawab Khan joined the Indian Army when he was only thirteen years old and served in the first Sudan War of 1882-1883. His other campaigns included Burma (1885-1893), the Chatral Frontier (1893-1896), the South African Anglo-Boer War (1899-1902), and the Zulu Rebellion of 1906. As a result of his leading role in the Satyagraha movement, Captain Khan lost his grant of land and his pension was terminated. He died on 11 August 1939, aged eighty. The old soldier was buried in unmarked grave number 1404 in the Muslim section.

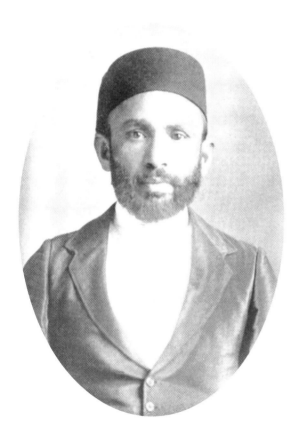

**Staunch resistance leader,
Ahmed Mohammed Cachalia**

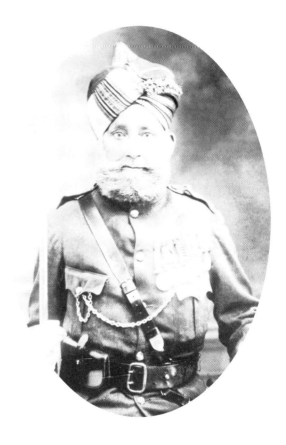

**Captain Jamadar Nawab Khan
of the Indian Army**

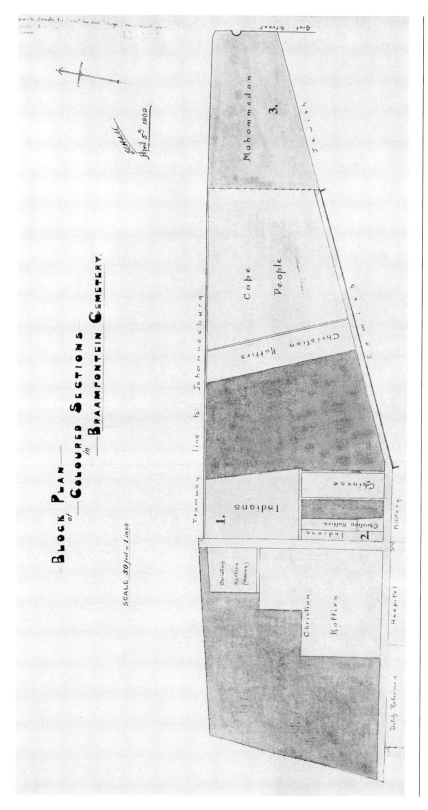

The elaborately segregated 'non-white' cemetery in Braamfontein, showing the grave sites of Nagappen (1), Valliamma (2) and A M Cachalia (3)

WESTERN
DISTRICTS

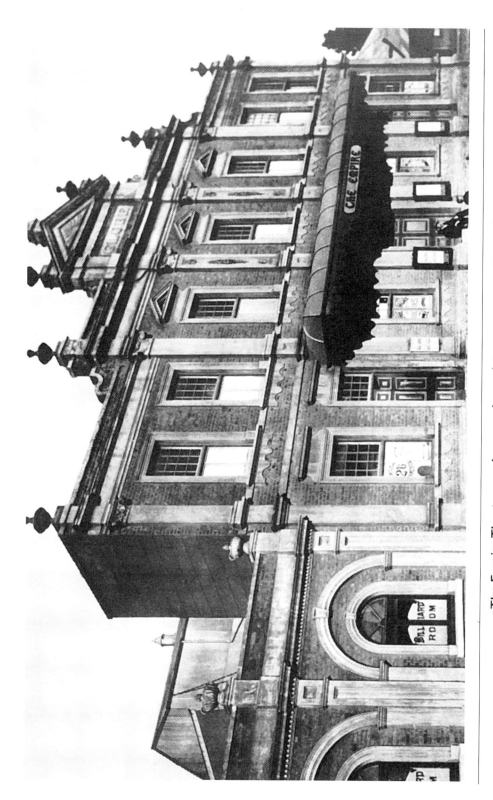

The Empire Theatre ... where passive resistance announced its arrival

EMPIRE THEATRE

Corner Commissioner and Ferreira Streets.
Ferreira House now covers the site.

THERE were two Empire Theatres in early Johannes-burg, both of which have disappeared.[56] The first was built in the late 1880s at the corner of Commissioner and Ferreira Streets, near the original centre of the mining camp. The second was a much grander building at the corner of Kruis and Commissioner Streets.

The passive resistance movement was launched at the historic mass meeting chaired by Gandhi at the first Empire Theatre on 11 September 1906. More than 3 000 people (including a Chinese delegation) angrily rejected the Transvaal Asiatic Law Amendment Ordinance. The *Rand Daily Mail* recognised it as one of the most remarkable meetings seen in Johannesburg.

The size of the meeting, the enthusiasm of the audience – practically the entire Indian population ceased to work for the day – and the depth of feeling displayed, formed a striking testimony to the indignation which the proposed legislation has aroused.[57]

The Ordinance which had provoked this furious reaction required Asians of eight years old or more to carry passes and register for them by giving fingerprints; enforced their segregation for residence and trade; and not only excluded new Asian immigration to the Transvaal, but threatened the rights of those who had lived there before the Anglo-Boer War and had left temporarily during the War.

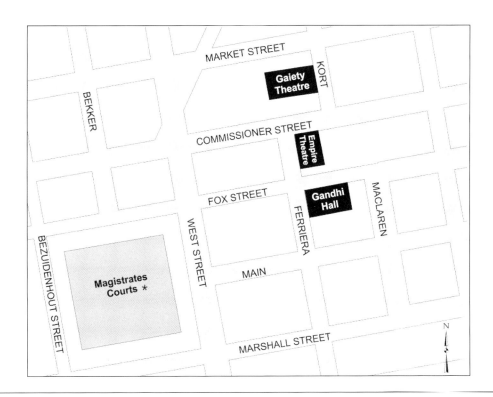

Gandhi sites on the outskirts of town: The early Gaiety and Empire Theatres and the more recent Gandhi Hall. The present Magistrates Courts opened in 1936, taking over from Johannesburg's first courts on Government Square

The meeting adopted an oath committing Indians to oppose these injustices even if it meant imprisonment. The famous Fourth Resolution states that should the Ordinance not be removed:

> *… this mass meeting of British Indians here assembled, solemnly and regretfully resolves that, rather than submit to the galling, tyrannous and un-British requirements laid down in the above draft Ordinance, every British Indian in the Transvaal shall submit himself to imprisonment, and shall continue so to do until it shall please His Most Gracious Majesty the King-Emperor to grant relief.*[58]

That night, Henry Polak records, the original Empire Theatre was destroyed by an accidental fire[59] but, in the words of prominent Pretoria Satyagrahi Gaurishankar Vyas at a meeting at the Gaiety on 29 March 1907, 'though the theatre was gutted by fire, the words spoken there live on'.[60]

GAIETY THEATRE
3 Kort Street, on the eastern side of the block now occupied by the Southern Life Centre.

THE GAIETY served as a theatre from the 1890s to the late 1920s, mostly as a venue for the great actor-manager of the time, Leonard Rayne. Gandhi's connection with the theatre was highlighted by newspaper columnist Percy Baneshik in 1983:

> *At a point in the 1910s when the playhouse was otherwise in the doldrums, it became the scene of a mass meeting of Transvaal Indians who heard Gandhi exhorting them to burn their pass documents. Which they did, there and then.*[61]

The report appears to have conflated several different meetings. The major Indian pass burning protests took place in August 1908 at a mosque in Newtown, and not at a theatre. Baneshik does not give a date for the meeting he describes or reveal the source of

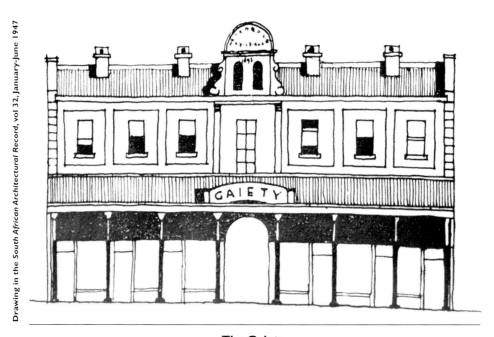

Drawing in the *South African Architectural Record*, vol 32, January-June 1947

The Gaiety

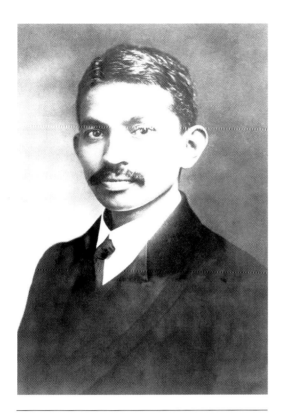

M K Gandhi in 1906, the year passive resistance was launched

his information. Fortunately, Gandhi's participation in other meetings at the Gaiety is better documented.

On 29 March 1907 Gandhi attended a huge meeting of Transvaal Indians who protested against the Asiatic Registration Act and offered voluntary registration. Delegates from all over the Transvaal converged on the small theatre near the western edge of town. Many had to leave, as the theatre was filled to capacity. On 4 April Gandhi called on Smuts in Pretoria and presented the resolutions adopted at the Gaiety.[62]

Gandhi served his final term of imprisonment in South Africa in 1913. After his release from Pretoria Central Prison on that occasion, he travelled to Johannesburg and addressed a mass meeting at the Gaiety on the evening of 18 December. *Indian Opinion* reported him as saying:

He [Gandhi] was not in the least thankful for having been released, for he preferred solitude and the peace of prison because it gave him opportunity and time for meditation; but, having been released, he should now resume the work upon which he was engaged when he was convicted.[63]

On 13 July 1914, a few days before he left Johannesburg and South Africa forever, Gandhi was back at the Gaiety to address a meeting. At last, he told his audience, a settlement had been reached that was honourable to both sides, and in keeping with the dignity of passive resisters.[64] It was with a sense of a mission fulfilled that he took leave of the country.

The Indian Relief Act of 1914 brought the curtain down on Satyagraha. Although his people had not won their freedom, Gandhi could claim a partial victory. The new law did not address all Indian grievances, but it did offer some concessions.

GANDHI HALL
Corner of Fox and Ferreira Streets. The site, comprising stands 39, 40 and 41, is covered by 954 Marshalltown at the corner (formerly a Nedbank branch) and Protea House at 50 Fox Street.

ALTHOUGH it was erected in 1940, long after Gandhi left South Africa, Gandhi Hall is part of his legacy in more than name alone. During the apartheid era the hall provided a link with past struggles and was a symbol of the Gandhian tradition.

The Indian community continued to revere Gandhi, both for his exploits in South Africa and for his role in India's independence struggle. The Transvaal Hindu Seva Samaj organised special prayer meetings when his health deteriorated from fasting

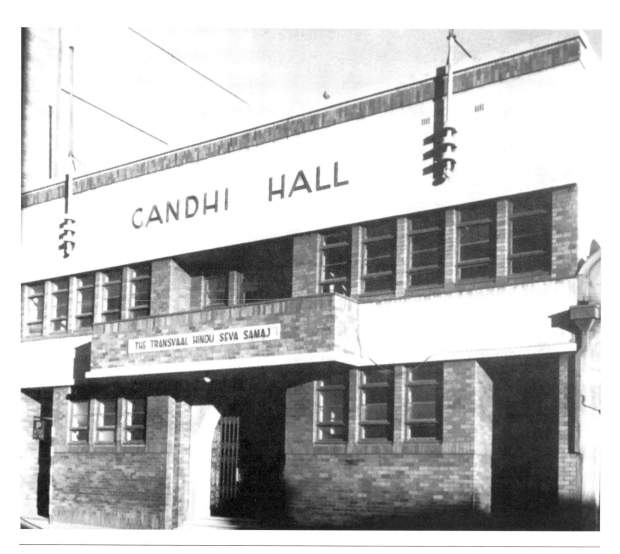

Gandhi Hall, a symbol of the Gandhian tradition for more than forty years in defiance of the British government in India. Gandhi Jayanti (birthday celebrations) were also held in the auditorium, in which large pictures of Gandhi and Nehru were displayed.

Gandhi Hall was built by the Transvaal Hindu Seva Samaj, a community organisation formed in 1932.[65] At that time, Johannesburg's Hindu community had no hall of its own and the establishment of one became one of the Samaj's earliest priorities. In October 1933, just eighteen months after the inception of the Samaj, the organisation acquired the necessary land in Marshalltown on leasehold. The location – across the road from the old Empire Theatre site – could hardly have been more appropriate. The Samaj appointed Hermann Kallenbach, by then a partner in the firm Kallenbach, Kennedy and Furner, as its architect. Kallenbach gave his services free of charge, and the plans were completed in 1939.

Ambaram Billimoria, who was President of the Samaj when the construction contract was awarded, had spent time as a boy with Gandhi on Tolstoy Farm. Other leading figures in the organisation were former comrades of Gandhi. Naran Patel, a Vice-President of the Samaj during the 1930s, had been imprisoned as a passive resister and was a former Vice-President of the Transvaal British Indian Association. Surendra Medh, another veteran Satyagrahi, was also prominent in the Samaj. During the Zulu resistance of 1906 Medh had been a sergeant in the Stretcher-bearer Corps established by Gandhi. By late 1913 he had been jailed eleven times as a passive resister, and been imprisoned for longer than any of his comrades.[66]

Gandhi Hall was one of the few auditoriums near the city centre which was open to racially integrated audiences. Not only were traditional Hindu festivals celebrated there, it was used for civic functions and political meetings. The African National Congress, Transvaal Indian Congress and other anti-apartheid organisations met at the hall, and it became identified with their struggle.

Under apartheid the site became part of a white 'group area'. The members of the community which used the hall were increasingly forced to move to Lenasia, an Indian 'group area' about 20 kilometres south-west of Johannesburg. As a result, the Marshalltown property was sold off in the mid-1980s. Money from the sale was used to build another Gandhi Hall in Impala Crescent, Section 5, Lenasia.[67]

At the Samaj's request, a brass plaque was erected at the entrance to Protea House. The inscription read:

Gandhi Hall
This property was built
on the stands on which the
Transvaal Hindu Seva Samaj
built a Hall in 1939 and named
it The Gandhi Hall to honour
the great Indian leader
Mahatma Gandhi (1869-1948)
who developed and evolved
during his stay in South Africa
(1893-1914)
the principles of Satyagraha

Sadly, the small plaque has disappeared, carried away early in 1999 to be recycled by one of Johannesburg's many unscrupulous dealers in scrap metal.

TRANSVAAL CHINESE ASSOCIATION HEADQUARTERS

2 Marshall Street, Ferreirastown. The Supa Quick company now has a storeroom on this site.

THE CHINESE pledged support for the Fourth Resolution adopted at the Empire Theatre meeting of 1906. As Asiatics, the Chinese united with Indians in the common cause of opposition to the new Ordinance and the anti-Asian legislation that followed. Many Chinese passive resisters went willingly to jail, sacrificed their livelihoods and even faced deportation from the Transvaal.[68]

The majority of Johannesburg's tiny population of free Chinese (as distinct from indentured miners) lived and worked in Ferreirastown – an area bounded by Commissioner, Alexander, Ferreira and Frederik Streets. Here they established their first social clubs and political organisations.

Chinese passive resistance was led by the Transvaal Chinese Association (TCA), at that time the major representative Chinese body. The Association was founded in 1903 and reached its peak by 1908.

When passive resistance came to an end for the Chinese in 1911 the Association was in sharp decline and was virtually a spent force.

In November 1907 TCA Chairman, Leung Quinn, invited Gandhi to address a memorial service for Chow Kwai For, a Chinese who, feeling degraded because he had submitted to registration, committed suicide.

A traditional funeral service was held at the Association's headquarters in Marshall Street on 27 November. Chinese inscriptions were hung on the walls of the spacious hall and a portrait of Chow, painted on silk, was placed over an altar of flowers and burning sandalwood.

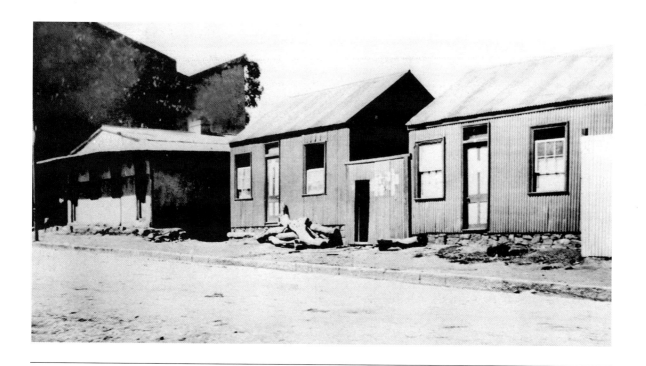

The Chinese Quarter: Typical dwellings in Ferreirastown

Gandhi described the scene:

No one present ... could help feeling admiration for the Chinese. Their beautiful hall was adorned with black cloth. On one side in the hall there was a photograph of the Chinaman who had died. In the centre were standing all those who had served as pickets. Surrounding them on all sides were chairs which were occupied by invitees. About a thousand Chinese, with flowers in their hands, gently passed by the photograph, praying for the soul of the departed one and went out through the door opposite. Then they sang dirges in Chinese ... Their unity, neatness and courage – all these things deserve to be emulated by us.[69]

A year after Chow's death, the Chinese community erected a tombstone on his grave which is behind that of Valliamma, in the Chinese section at Braamfontein Cemetery.

Gandhi and other Indian leaders addressed numerous gatherings of the Chinese Association, and Chinese were often present at Indian mass meetings. Nevertheless the two groups maintained their own organisations and independence. Underlining this, Gandhi wrote in later years:

Still from first to last the activities of the two communities were not allowed to be mixed up. Each worked through its own independent organisation. This arrangement produced the beneficent result that so long as both the communities stood to their guns, each would be a source of strength to the other. But if one of the two gave way, that would leave the morale of the other unaffected or at least the other would steer clear of the danger of a total collapse.[70]

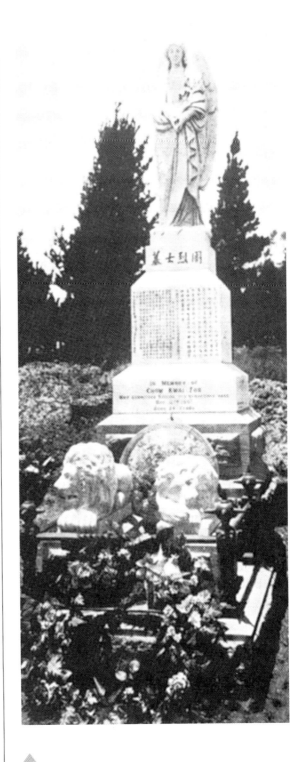

Tombstone honouring Chow Kwai For, 'Who committed suicide for conscience sake'

47

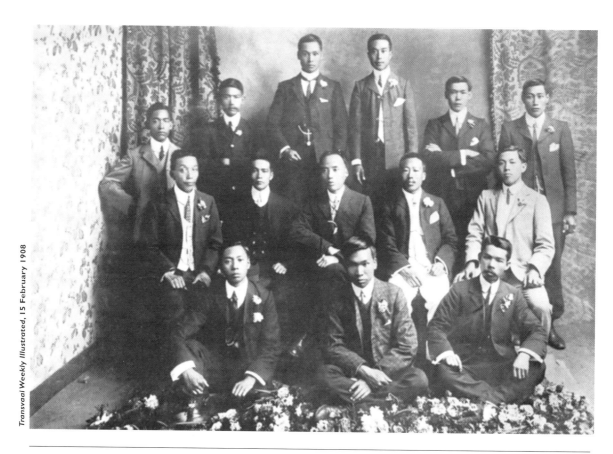

Transvaal Weekly Illustrated, 15 February 1908

Chinese passive resisters. Leung Quinn, Chairman of the Transvaal Chinese Association, is in the centre

CANTONESE CLUB

1 Fox Street, at the corner of Alexander Street, Ferreirastown. A furniture workshop now marks this site.

THE CANTONESE CLUB dates from the 1890s and is the oldest known Chinese organisation in Johannesburg. Gandhi's ally, Leung Quinn, was Chairman for a number of years, and the Club became known as a centre of passive resistance. In more recent times the Club has often harked back to its role in the struggle. A membership certificate issued in 1919 states (inaccurately) that the club was only established in 1908 to resist the unjust law, and that its core consisted of members known as the passive resistance party.[71]

The building which housed the Club stood in the heart of the Chinese district. The two-storey building included various games rooms and a large hall used for weddings, parties and funerals. Sleeping accommodation was available for rent. Gandhi was quick to point out that similar accommodation was also needed in the Indian community. As he knew only too well, white hoteliers seldom welcomed non-white guests.

Gandhi regarded the Cantonese Club as a model community centre. In 1905, the year club members erected their Fox Steet clubhouse, he challenged readers of *Indian Opinion* to emulate their example:

The Cantonese Club in 1955 ▶

Since the Chinese have no facilities for lodging, they have started a Cantonese Club, which serves as a meeting place, a lodge and also as a library. They have acquired for the Club land on a long lease and have built on it a pucca one-storeyed building. There they all live in great cleanliness and do not stint themselves in the matter of living space; and seen within and from the outside, it would look like some good European Club. They have in it separate rooms marked drawing, dining, meeting, committee room and the Secretary's room and the library, and do not use any room except for the purpose for which it is intended. Other rooms adjoining these are let out as bedrooms. It is such a fine and clean place that any Chinese gentleman visiting the town can be put up there. The entrance fee is £5, and the annual subscription varies according to the member's profession. The Club has about 150 members who meet every Sunday and amuse themselves with games. The members can avail themselves of club facilities on week days also.

We have nothing similar to boast of. In no city of South Africa have we a place of our own where an Indian visitor can be put up. Our hospitality is no doubt excellent, but it is bound to be limited. … It is up to us to take a lesson from the Club founded by the Chinese and start one on the same pattern.[72]

Fire caused extensive damage to the clubhouse in the late 1940s. Major renovations followed and the building was modernised. The Cantonese Club remained a focal point in the Chinese area until the early 1980s when the building was finally demolished.[73]

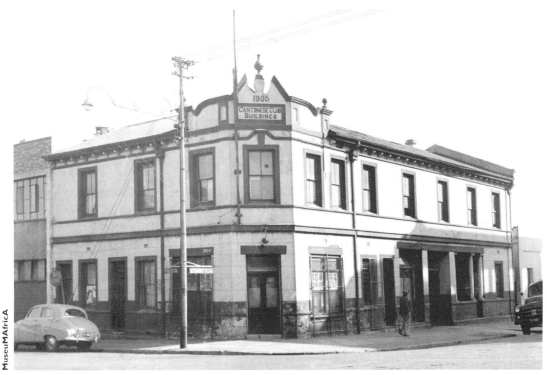

MuseuMAfricA

INDIAN LOCATION, NEWTOWN

Bounded by Carr Street (north side), Malherbe Street (west), Goch Street (east, under M1 highway), and Pim Street (south).

NEWTOWN'S 'Coolie Location' was established in 1887 as Johannesburg's first Indian settlement. In fact, it did not house Indians alone, and when the location was evacuated in March 1904 its population comprised 1 642 Indians, 1 420 Africans and 146 'Cape Coloureds'. [74] Albert West described how the area had been allowed to degenerate into a slum:

> *The Indian Location in Johannesburg was in a deplorable condition, being without proper roads, lighting or sanitation, the dilapidated buildings being mostly of wood or iron. The residents acquired their plots on a lease of ninety-nine years. People were densely packed together, the area of which never increased with the increase of population. Beyond arranging to clear the latrines in a haphazard way, the municipality did nothing to provide any sanitary facilities.*[75]

In 1904, after an outbreak of bubonic plague, the Indian Location was burnt to the ground by the authorities and the entire population was removed to an emergency camp near the sewerage works at Klipspruit (later Pimville), thirteen miles south of Johannesburg. The origins of Soweto, Johannesburg's sprawling dormitory township for Africans, go back to the evacuation camp at Klipspruit.

TEMPORARY PLAGUE HOSPITAL

76 Carr Street, Newtown. A Premier Milling plant now covers the site.

THE WORST epidemic of bubonic plague in Johannesburg's history struck the Indian Location in 1904. Gandhi had repeatedly warned the Town Council that its neglect of overcrowding and squalor in the area could lead to such an epidemic. The Municipality failed to heed the warnings, and in March 1904 plague spread to the location from a gold mine where some Indians worked.

On 18 March Gandhi received an alarming note from Madanjit Vyavaharik, the publisher of *Indian*

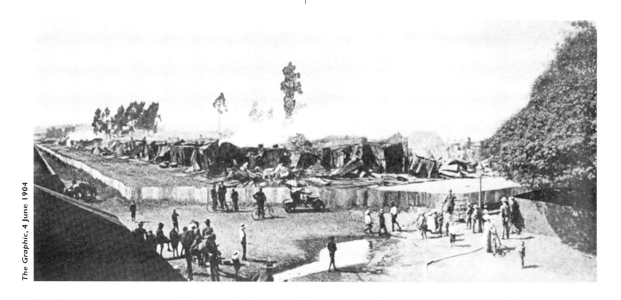

The Graphic, 4 June 1904

The burning of Newtown's 'Coolie Location'

Opinion who had been in the location, canvassing subscribers for the newspaper. Madanjit informed him that Indians were dying in the location. Together with four Indian volunteers (Gandhi selected young, unmarried men because of the risk), and Madanjit, Gandhi took swift and decisive action to care for the sick and arrest the spread of disease.

Dr William Godfrey, also an Indian, soon joined them. Madanjit broke the lock on a vacant house on Stand 36[76], and this was used as an isolation and treatment hospital. During the evening of 18 March Gandhi and his co-workers obtained beds and blankets, and removed plague victims to Stand 36. They nursed and fed fourteen patients, making them as comfortable as was possible in the small, overcrowded rooms.

The makeshift hospital was on Locatie (now Carr) Street, which led to the railway station and was lined with shops and eating houses.[77] Across the road, and just outside the Indian Location's northern boundary, was a railway compound for African workers dating from the late 1890s. The compound building has survived, and now houses Bezekela College. A total of 112 people contracted plague, and eighty-two died. Gandhi described the suffering and loss of life he had witnessed:

The victims again, have been carried away in an incredibly short time. What at first appeared to be a slight fever and a little coughing, in a few hours or the second day, developed into high fever, spitting of blood, and violent paroxysms. The suffering of the patient is terrible. Delirium and death followed the third day. During the last stages, the patient gets so exhausted that, even though one notices intense agony on his face, the poor sufferer is not able to give it speech.[78]

On 20 March the Town Council finally reacted to the crisis by providing a large warehouse near the gas works as a temporary hospital. All the inhabitants of the Indian Location were removed to the tent camp on 30 March. A day later the entire location was put to flame by the Council. The destruction of the Indian Location, Gandhi believed, achieved an objective of the municipality. They had used the insanitary conditions caused by their own neglect as a pretext for removing an unwanted residential area.[79]

By October 1904 the area had been renamed Newtown and would be redeveloped as a commercial zone in which vast fortunes would be made in milling, produce, sugar and food merchandising.

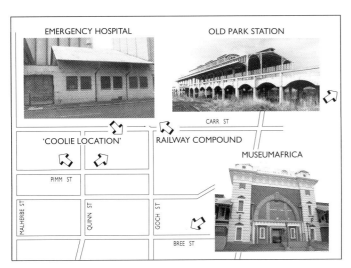

1. MUSEUMAFRICA
   This former fruit and vegetable market was the biggest building in South Africa when it was completed in 1913

2. 'COOLIE LOCATION'
   Johannesburg's first Indian settlement, burnt down by the Municipality in 1904

3. EMERGENCY HOSPITAL
   Here Gandhi nursed plague victims. Premier Milling built on this site in 1913-1914

4. RAILWAY COMPOUND
   Housed African workers from the 1890s

5. OLD PARK STATION
   Moved to Newtown in 1986

Northern Newtown

OLD PARK STATION
Formerly in Eloff Street, now reassembled in Northern Newtown, off Carr Street.

THE MAIN building of the old Park Station, Johannesburg's major railway station from 1897 to 1952, was imported from Holland in 1896. The elegant cast-iron and glass building was erected in 1897 on a site bordered by Rissik Street in the west and Hoek Street in the east. In 1952 the old building made way for the present Park Station in 1952. The structure was dismantled and rebuilt at Transnet's Esselen Park Training Centre where it remained until 1986, when the old station canopy was reassembled in Newtown, immediately south of the Braamfontein Railway Yard, and close to where it had stood in Gandhi's time.[80]

Gandhi was a familiar figure on the platforms of the station. He became a frequent commuter, especially between Johannesburg and Durban. He met delegations there and was met himself. He often alighted from trains to a hero's welcome, with the station decorated in his honour. Olive Doke, the Rev Joseph Doke's daughter, wrote that:

> *Great welcomes were given to Mr. Gandhi on his arrival back at Park Station, after having been away on behalf of the cause, or else on the arrival of distinguished visitors. Flowers and garlands were always prominent on such occasions and made things very colourful as various friends received the honour of being garlanded, whilst the crowds surged around waving and articulating their welcome. These were historical days, and Mr. Gandhi in all his humility was the central figure.*[81]

Gandhi's arrival from Pretoria on 24 May 1909 was greeted by a thousand Indian and Chinese supporters.[82] Later that year an even bigger crowd

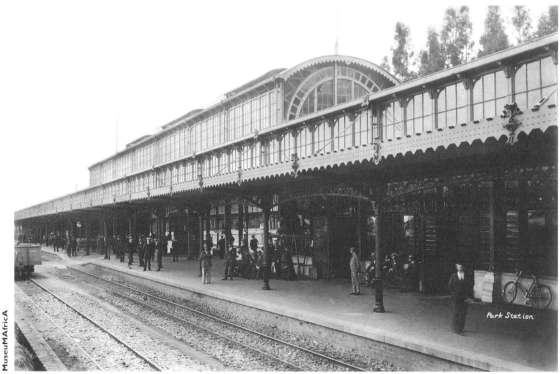

MuseuMAfricA

welcomed Gandhi and Hajee Habib, who comprised a deputation which had just returned from England. Two thousand Indians and Chinese were waiting when their train steamed in on 2 December.[83]

On 25 October 1908, Gandhi was also responsible for one of the most remarkable scenes to take place at Park Station when he was transferred from Volksrust Prison to the Fort. He stepped off the train under guard, wearing his prison uniform marked with broad arrows. Station officials and police looked on in amazement as supporters garlanded him with flowers. Henry Polak takes up the story:

> *The warder appeared to realise the incongruity of the situation, for he bore himself towards the prisoner with every reasonable mark of respect. For this was evidently a person of some importance, to whom a certain degree of deference must be shown. The subject of conversation was whether the prisoner preferred to go by cab or to walk to the jail. If the former, he would have to pay for it. He, however, declined the easier way, and being a practised and easy walker, he chose to march the three-quarters of a mile, in broad daylight in his convict suit. Resolutely shouldering his bag, he stepped out smartly, we shamefacedly following at a respectful distance.*[84]

◁ Park Station in the early 1900s

HAMIDIA MOSQUE (ALSO KNOWN AS THE FORDSBURG MOSQUE AND THE NEWTOWN MOSQUE)
2 Jennings Street, Newtown.

INDIANS in the Transvaal were divided along language, class, caste and religious lines. Gandhi used his influence and personal example to promote mutual respect, unity in action and co-operation between Hindus and Muslims. He collaborated closely with the leading Muslim organisation in the Transvaal, the Hamidia Islamic Society, which had been established in Johannesburg in July 1906 for the social welfare of Muslims. The Society was named after Sultan Abdul Hamid of the Ottoman Empire who, in 1909, was deposed by Young Turks.

An organisation comprising mainly Muslim merchants, the Society used passive resistance tactics to oppose racial discrimination and injustice. By the end of 1907, it had several hundred members. Its mass meetings, held on Sundays at the grounds of the Newtown Mosque, attracted large crowds of merchants and workers.[85]

As a non-Muslim, Gandhi could not hold an official leadership position in the Society, but he often addressed its meetings.

A report in *The Star* describes an impromptu meeting called by Gandhi on 10 January 1908:

> *… Mr. Gandhi and other Indians and Chinese who were ordered to leave the Colony within 48 hours a fortnight ago were called upon to attend Court for sentence. There was a large gathering outside B Court at ten o clock, and before the doors were opened word was circulated that the proceedings against the defaulters would not be taken until the afternoon. Mr. Gandhi availed himself of the opportunity the few hours postponement*

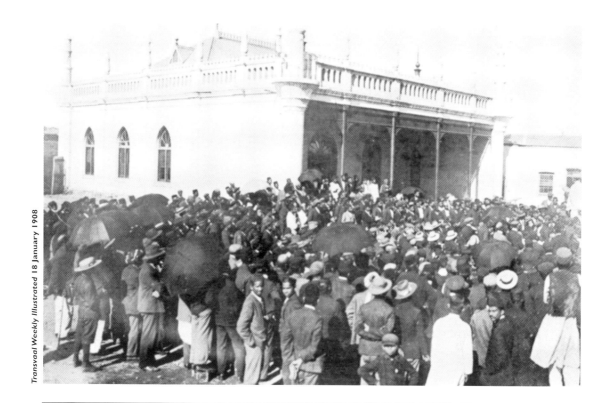

Mass meeting outside the Hamidia Mosque

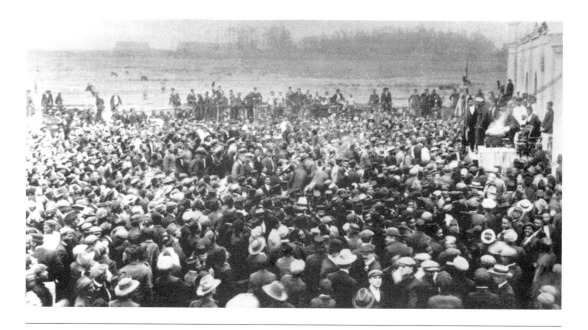

Registration certificates go up in flames outside the mosque

allowed to address his countrymen. It was to be a valedictory exhortation to the rank and file of the Indians to stand firm during the incarceration of the leaders of the passive resisters movement. The meeting was held in the Mosque grounds, Newtown, at 11 o'clock, and despite the short notice of the meeting there was a large gathering. For the purpose of such [a] meeting a platform had been erected in the grounds, and seating accommodation was provided by means of the serviceable paraffin tins which were strewn about in thousands. On the platform were Essop Ismail Mia, Chairman of the British Indian Association, an Indian priest in an artistic Oriental garb, and Mr. Gandhi. A few introductory remarks were made by Mr. Mia, and then Mr. Gandhi spoke. He was listened to with great intentness. Every eye was fixed upon the slim central figure of Mr. Gandhi, and the meeting gave an indication of the hold he has upon his countrymen.[86]

The burning of voluntary registration certificates at the mosque grounds kick-started the resumption of Satyagraha in August 1908. Gandhi called on Indians to burn their certificates only after the Transvaal government turned away appeals for compromise. He told the government that 'If the Asiatic Act is not repealed in terms of the settlement, and if the Government's decision to that effect is not communicated before a specific date, the certificates collected will be burnt, and we will humbly take the consequences.'[87]

More than 3 000 Indians gathered outside the mosque two hours after the expiry of the time limit on 16 August 1908, to perform the public ceremony of burning the certificates. As the meeting was about to begin, a volunteer arrived on a bicycle with a telegram announcing the government's refusal to repeal the hated Act.

The news was read to the assembly, who greeted it with loud cheers. More than 1 200 certificates were thrown into a big cauldron, doused with paraffin, and set alight.

Among those present at the meeting was Mir Alam Khan. Gandhi picks up the story:

Mir Alam … announced that he had done wrong to assault me as he did, and to the great joy of the audience, handed his original certificate to be burnt, as he had not taken a voluntary certificate. I took hold of his hand, pressed it with joy, and assured him once more that I never harboured in my mind any resentment against him.[88]

The crowd which massed at the mosque grounds for the follow-up meeting of 23 August was, if anything, even bigger than that of the week before. After Gandhi's speech another 525 certificates were burned.

PAGEVIEW
Bounded by 11th Street (north side), Krause Street (west), De La Rey Street (east) and 23rd Street (south).

PAGEVIEW became an important centre of the Indian community after the Indian Location was burned down. From the 1890s to 1904 the area was known as Malay Location, and the population was mainly 'coloured' and 'Malay'. The shift to a predominantly Indian population began around June 1904 when people evacuated from Newtown moved back to the urban centre. Most of the displaced Indians settled in Malay Location, one of the very few areas available in Johannesburg for legal 'non-white' occupation.[89]

Conditions in Pageview contrasted sharply with those of the insanitary shacks of Newtown. Writing just a fortnight before plague struck Newtown, Gandhi describes Malay Location as a flourishing place:

> There never has been even so much as a whisper against the place from a sanitary standpoint. The residents live very decently. They have built substantial premises; some of them have built even brick buildings.[90]

HAMIDIA HALL
Number 10 17th Street, Pageview.

A SMALL HALL in Pageview became a nerve centre of early passive resistance. Indian leaders held crucial talks there in September 1906 during the week preceding the public meeting at the Empire Theatre. According to Gandhi, all the leading Indians held consultations at these meetings, which laid the groundwork for the watershed meeting at the theatre.[91]

Hamidia Hall was heavily used by both organisations at the forefront of Indian resistance in the Transvaal – the British Indian Association and the Hamidia Islamic Society. Gandhi founded the British Indian Association in 1903 and became its Secretary and chief strategist. As the Association had no hall of its own, it often met at Hamidia Hall, and used mosque grounds in Fordsburg and Pretoria for large public demonstrations.[92]

Hamidia Hall, was on 17th Street[93], now a busy thoroughfare. It was one of only a few halls in Pageview during the early 20th century and was later converted into a cinema. During the 1960s it was known as the Avalon.[94] By the 1970s it had been renamed the Taj[95] and tended to specialise in Indian films.[96] Some of the Taj's patrons were still familiar with local traditions linking the hall to Gandhi and passive resistance.[97] Like many of Pageview's other landmarks, the Hamidia Hall has long since disappeared.

HINDU CREMATORIUM
Coloured Section, Brixton Cemetery (western end).

IN EARLY Johannesburg most Hindus were forced to contravene their own religious beliefs by burying their dead. No facilities were readily available for cremation and the last rites according to the Hindu religion.

After moving to the town in 1906, the builder Narandas Damania discussed the need for a crematorium with leaders of the Hindu community. In 1908 Messrs Damania, Ghelani and Tekchand approached Gandhi to help obtain suitable land for a crematorium.[98]

Gandhi negotiated with the Town Council on behalf of the Hindu community and through his efforts, the land on which the crematorium stands was set aside for them. The edifice was built free of charge by Narandas Damania, who, in 1910, was also to make an important contribution at Tolstoy Farm where he declined to charge and convinced other artisans to work at reduced rates. [99]

The proposed crematorium was discussed at a meeting of the Town Council on 24 September 1912. The minutes of the meeting record the discussion as follows:

> For some time past we have had under consideration the question of allocating a suitable piece of ground for the erection of a Hindoo Crematorium. There has been a certain amount of doubt as to whether, in the

event of the Council agreeing to the erection of the Hindoo Crematorium, it might not be necessary to grant sites to other sects for the establishment of crematoria. Following on this we have interviewed Mr. Gandhi with regard to the whole question. It has been pointed out that the Hindoo Committee, which is the responsible body, would be willing to allow other sects to cremate if desired, and any charges which might be imposed would be submitted to the Council for approval. Although according to the religious rites of Hindoos, the remains of any body are not buried, but taken away by the mourners in small receptacles provided for the purpose, it was represented that as much ground as possible should be allocated to the crematorium.[100]

The meeting recommended that a portion of ground 75x50 feet in extent, in the Coloured Section of Brixton Cemetery, be allocated for a Hindu Crematorium.

Gandhi commissioned Hermann Kallenbach to draw up plans. These later disappeared from the offices of the British Indian Association and had to be redrawn.[101]

It would be five years before the Hindu Community was able to take advantage of the Council's offer. A Crematorium Committee was formed to collect the necessary funds but it had little success and eventually called a general meeting of the community under Gandhi's chairmanship. Despite Gandhi's plea for donations, there was little forthcoming as most of those who attended the meeting were labourers with small incomes. Not until 1917 had sufficient money had been raised. The community felt that the area set aside by the Council was too small, and asked for a site measuring 150x150 feet. Council agreed to this request in May 1917, and the crematorium was built the following year. A new gas-fired crematorium was built in 1956 to replace the original wood-burning one.

The old crematorium is adjacent to the new one, in a large walled precinct. From a Hindu religious point of view the original crematorium should never be demolished.

The Hindu Crematorium is administered by the Hindu Crematorium Committee, a sub-committee of the Hindu Seva Samaj. In 1993 the Crematorium Committee asked the National Monuments Council to declare the old crematorium a national monument. This was done officially on 22 September 1995. The English inscription on the plaque erected at the site by the National Monuments Council reads:

HINDU CREMATORIUM

This structure, erected in 1918, was the first brick-built crematorium in Africa.
M K Gandhi, acting as lawyer for the Hindu community, obtained suitable land for the crematorium. Many donations were received from both rural and urban areas in the Transvaal. The crematorium, built by Messrs Damania and Kalidas, is a fine example of decorative brickwork.
National Monuments Council
Declared 1995[102]

RANGERS FOOTBALL GROUND
Arthur Bloch Park, Mayfair

A GROUP of miners from Newcastle, England, and Glasgow, Scotland, founded Rangers Football Club in 1889. The Club's inaugural meeting was held in a house on the border between Fordsburg and Crown Mines.[103] Although Arthur Bloch Park was primarily the home of the Rangers Club, it was known to be open to all comers and football pitches there still attract Indian teams from Mayfair and surrounding areas.

From about 1910 to 1913 Gandhi promoted passive resisters' soccer matches at the Rangers Ground. Together with Lewis Ritch, he addressed a crowd after a match on 5 June 1911. In the company of Tolstoy Farm's schoolboys, Gandhi also attended a match on 23 September 1911.[104]

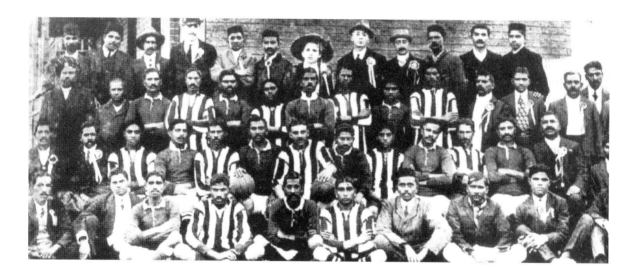

Pretoria Passive Resisters (striped jerseys) played against Johannesburg Passive Resisters at the Rangers Ground in May 1911. Gandhi is sixth from the left in the back row

IN THE
SUBURBS

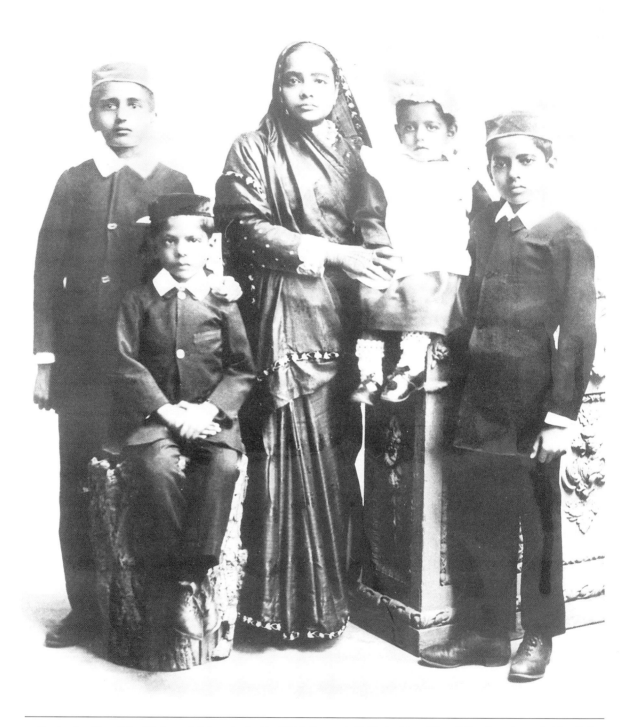

Kasturba Gandhi with her children in India, 1898. From left: Gokuldas (Gandhi's sister's son), Manilal (seated), Kasturba Gandhi, Ramdas and Harilal

11 ALBERMARLE STREET, TROYEVILLE

THOUGH his Indian constituency was concentrated in western Johannesburg, after the arrival of his family from India late in 1904, Gandhi moved to the Albermarle Street house at the eastern limit of the city, on the border of Troyeville and Kensington.

The rental was arranged by Charles Kew, the estate agent who had found Gandhi his office accommodation in Rissik Street. Kew wrote to Gandhi in October 1947 recalling how Troyeville residents had tried to keep Gandhi out of their whites-only suburb. Displaying 'considerable indignation,' writes Kew, 'they tried before you took possession to offset the tendency but the owner of the house supported me, and in a few weeks the agitation died down'.

Gandhi and his family – his wife Kasturba and their three sons, Manilal, aged twelve, Ramdas, aged nine and six-year-old Devdas – shared the house with Henry Polak as well as an Englishman, described by Millie Polak as 'engaged in the telegraph service' and a young Indian ward of Gandhi's.[105] Polak's wife, Millie Graham, joined them in 1905 having arrived from England on 30 December and married Polak the same day, with Gandhi as best man. The marriage certificate makes it clear that they were living in Albermarle Street, but no street number is stated.

Millie Polak, in her memoirs, described Gandhi's house:

The house was situated in a fairly good middle-class neighbourhood, on the outskirts of town. It was a double-storied, detached, eight-roomed building of the modern villa type, surrounded by a garden, and having, in front, the open spaces of the kopjes. The upstairs verandah was roomy enough to sleep on it, if one wished to do so, and, indeed, in warm weather, it was often so used.[106]

It has long been thought that Millie was describing the house at 19 Albermarle Street. Wishful thinking helped cement the association between Gandhi and Troyeville's most exotic home, with its curved balconies and suggestions of Oriental splendour. For many people the urge to superimpose the larger-than-life Indian leader onto this remarkable house proved irresistible. After buying the house in 1991 architect Michael Hart tried to establish that Gandhi had really lived there, and submitted his findings to the National Monuments Council. Number 19 was declared a national monument in 1994, partly because of its supposed value as a Gandhi site.

The house at Number 19 was designed by and built for the Swiss architect Eugene Metzler. As an example of European Art Nouveau in South Africa, built when the standard was Victorian colonial, the house is architecturally significant.[107] Metzler's house would, however, have been too ostentatious for Gandhi, whose emphasis on simplicity increased during this period.

Number 19's claim to be a Gandhi house has recently been challenged by Professor James Hunt,[108] a renowned scholar of Gandhi sites. As Hunt points out, the Metzler house was built too late for Gandhi to move in. Municipal records reveal that Metzler submitted plans for his house on 17 May 1905, and they were passed on 20 May. The foundations were only inspected on 15 March 1906. How long Metzler lived in the house is uncertain. But after the house was completed in 1906, there would hardly have been time for Gandhi to have stayed there.

The real Gandhi house in Troyeville is at Number 11 Albermarle Street, one block higher than Metzler's house. Also a double-storey with an upstairs

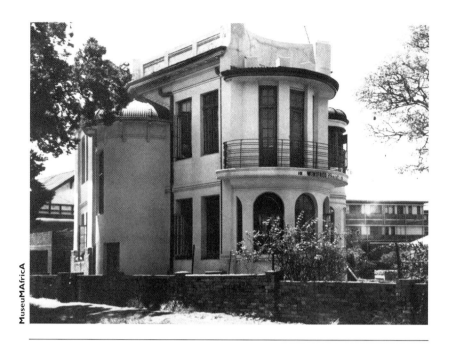

A national monument but not a Gandhi house, 19 Albermarle Street

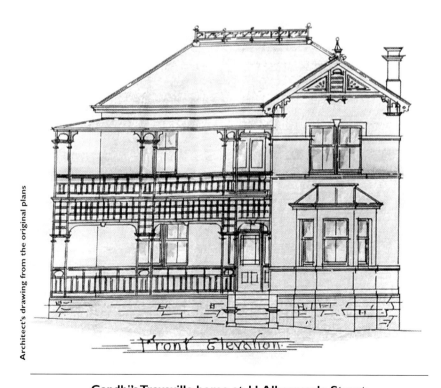

Front Elevation

Gandhi's Troyeville home at 11 Albermarle Street

balcony, Number 11 has a more conventional Victorian design. Mr J T Ellis submitted plans for the house on 7 July 1903, and they were approved on 10 July. As with Number 19, there is no record of the date when the building was completed, but the house was practically brand new when Gandhi began renting it around October 1904.

Hunt states the case for Number 11:

For me the evidence is clear, as we have the word from Manilal Gandhi himself. Born in 1892, he was twelve years old in 1904 and fourteen years old in 1906, so he would remember it well. In 1952 he took Dr Homer Jack [an American clergyman and Gandhian activist] to 11 Albermarle Street. Manilal, then sixty years old, walked through the house and recalled the people who were there and the events that took place in specific rooms. [109]

Their tour is recounted in Homer Jack's article, *In the footsteps of Mahatma Gandhi* (published in late 1952 or early 1953):

We went through the house, room by room, as Manilal pointed out the places where father and mother slept and how the house had not really changed much. … Manilal pointed to the alcove off the kitchen where the handmill stood and where 'Mr. Polak, father, and I would grind our own flour'. He told how the living room was used for a reception after Mr. Polak's marriage and how, when a painter dirtied all the walls while painting the ceiling, his father testily ordered the walls done within 24 hours.

In his article Dr Jack gives the address as '112 Albermarle', but his diary lists it correctly as Number 11, and gives the date of the visit: Saturday 12 July 1952. In the article it is mentioned that the Gandhi house 'turned out to be the parsonage of a Methodist missionary, and so we were well received'. Plans for additions to the house confirm that Number 11 was owned by the Wesleyan Methodist Missionary Society.

The Gandhis left Troyeville in May or June 1906, as a result of the Zulu resistance in Natal (the Bambatha Rebellion). Gandhi explained:

I thought I must do my bit in the war. With the community's permission, therefore, I made an offer to the Government to raise a Stretcher-bearer Corps for service with the troops. The offer was accepted. I therefore broke up my Johannesburg home and sent my family to Phoenix in Natal where my co-workers had settled and from where Indian Opinion *was published.* [110]

The family did not return to Albermarle Street. On 19 July 1906, after six weeks at the front, the Stretcher-bearer Corps was disbanded and Gandhi returned to Johannesburg without his wife and children. In August 1906 he moved into a small house near Highlands which he shared with the Polaks. [111]

SOUTH AFRICAN INDIAN WAR MONUMENT
At the summit of Observatory Ridge, north of Bezuidenhout Valley.

One of Johannesburg's first monuments honours British Indians who served on South African battlefields. Erected partly by public subscription in 1902, it stands as a memorial to Indians who died in the Anglo-Boer War of 1899-1902.

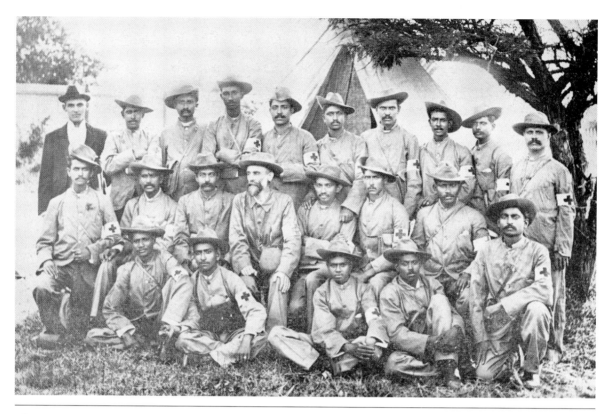

Gandhi raised a Stretcher-bearer Corps to serve in the Anglo-Boer War, 1899-1902. He is seated in the middle row, fifth from the left

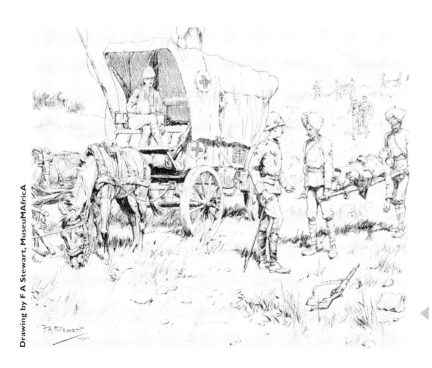

Indian stretcher bearers carrying the wounded to an ambulance wagon

A large contingent from the Indian Army was brought thousands of miles to reinforce British defences in Natal during the first year of the war. This force, consisting of three cavalry regiments, four infantry battalions, an ammunition column and a field hospital, made a major contribution to the British war effort. Besides the troops who came out in the first year, India supplied more than 7 000 non-combatants during the course of the war. They included transport men, water carriers, orderlies and washermen.

With persuasion from Gandhi, Indians who had already settled in South Africa offered their services too. Gandhi, at thirty-one, was a loyal British subject, and when war broke out he urged the local Indians to volunteer their services.

Despite having grave doubts about the justness of the British cause, Gandhi saw the war as an opportunity for Indians to prove their loyalty to the Empire. Indians should not only claim their rights as British subjects, he argued, but also do their duty as British subjects.

A formal offer of assistance was made by Gandhi but rejected by the Government. He made a second offer, emphasising the Indians' willingness to serve in any capacity, even as servants in hospitals. Again, the offer was rejected. But, with British losses mounting, permission was eventually given for the formation of an Indian Ambulance Corps.

About 1 000 stretcher bearers, mainly indentured Indians from Natal's sugar estates, went into the field. Their uniforms and supplies were provided by the Indian trading community. They were in action for seven days at the Battle of Colenso and were called up again about a month later for the Battle of Spioenkop, spending three weeks in the field and coming under fire more than once. Gandhi himself helped carry the dying General Woodgate[112] about twenty-five miles to the base hospital at Frere.[113]

Looking back on the war, Gandhi commented:

This contribution of the Indians in South Africa to the war was comparatively insignificant. They suffered hardly any loss of life. Yet a sincere desire to be of help is bound to impress the other party, and is doubly appreciated when it is quite unexpected. Such fine feeling for the Indians lasted during the continuance of the war.[114]

Indians did indeed enjoy new-found goodwill as a result of the war, if only for a short time. Major newspapers carried approving stories about Indian stretcher bearers – favourable press treatment which was a novel experience. But this 'fine feeling' evaporated soon after peace was declared.

The memorial is in the form of a large obelisk of sandstone cut from the ridge which it crowns. A tablet on the monument's east side bears the inscription:

To the memory of British Officers
Natives
NCOs and Men
Veterinary Assistants
Nalbands [water carriers]
and Followers of the Indian Army
Who died in South Africa.1899-1902

On the other three sides of the obelisk are tablets inscribed with the designations of the main religious groups involved:

'Mussulman [Muslim]',
'Christian – Zoroastrian',
'Hindu – Sikh'.

Indian Cemetery, Observatory Park.

Source: Property Register for Parks and Cemeteries

Indian Cemetery, Observatory Park

A photograph of the Indian monument was included as the only illustration in the first biography of Gandhi, Doke's *M K Gandhi: An Indian Patriot in South Africa*, published in 1909. The Rev Doke was at pains to place before British readers Gandhi's credentials as a loyal son of the Empire.

Over the years many people supposed that the memorial was intended for Gandhi's ambulance men. The fact that the tablets were unveiled while Gandhi was visiting India in 1902 suggests otherwise. Town Council minutes carry an invitation to a ceremony below the ridge:

Captain J.C.C. Perkins, the Native Officers, N.C.O.s and men of the Indian details, request the pleasure of the President and Members of the Johannesburg Municipality, their families and friends, to witness the unveiling of the Indian Monument at the Remount Depot, Bezuidenhout Valley, Johannesburg, by Lieut.-General the Hon. N.G. Lyttleton, K.C.B., commanding Transvaal and Orange River Colonies, at 3.45 p.m. on Friday, 31st October, 1902.[115]

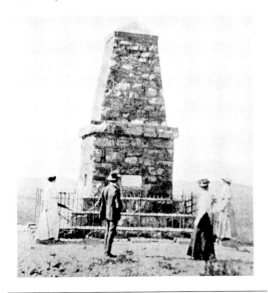

Monument to Indians in the Anglo-Boer War

About 4 000 horses could be accommodated at Bezuidenhout Valley's large central Remount Depot. The remount station was staffed by an Indian detachment, with four British officers, two veterinary surgeons and African assistants making up the rest of the establishment. The Indians, many of them Sikhs, were among the British forces which had occupied Johannesburg in 1900. Indian troops camped in what was to become Observatory Park, below the ridge on which the Indian monument was built. The campsite was chosen mainly for its abundant water – needed by both horses and men – supplied by springs which flowed throughout the year.

The Remount Depot was carelessly guarded and on 5 January 1901 news was received that Boer guerrillas planned to raid it. Steps were taken at once to reinforce the men on duty there, and the Boers presumably got wind of this as they made no move. Boers did, however, raid a remount depot at Braamfontein on 12 January, carrying off 512 horses. Then, early in February, Boers struck the Bezuidenhout Valley Remount Depot, taking all the serviceable horses.[116]

Four unknown Muslim soldiers were buried nearby in 1902, on the east side of the present Observatory Park, above the bowling greens.[117] The cause of their deaths is uncertain, though it is known that many of the Sikhs fell victim to typhus. A sandstone slab erected at the grave site by Captain Perkins, Indian Details, marks their burial place. The four bodies were exhumed when the municipality developed the park in 1964, making way for a Protea Garden. Their remains were reburied in Braamfontein Cemetery's Garden of Remembrance where a granite headstone is inscribed: 'Here lie the remains of four unknown Mohammedans who served as Indian details during the South African war and who were originally buried at Bezuidenhout Valley in August 1902'.

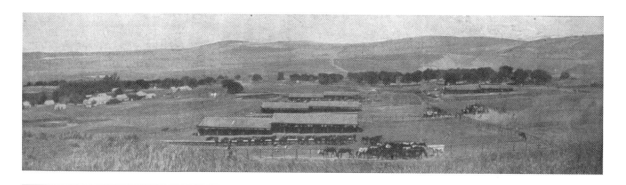

The British Army Remount Depot below Observatory Ridge

The memorial on Observatory Ridge has survived for nearly a century, defying vandals who have plagued much of its history. Within a year of being erected, the monument needed rescuing – the tablets were covered with scribbles and the fence was dilapidated. Acting swiftly, the municipality cleaned the tablets and informed the government that the monument was being defaced. After surrounding the monument with an unscaleable iron fence[118], the government handed the memorial over to the Town Council. Protection and maintenance of the monument – previously the government's responsibility – would henceforth be taken over by the municipality.

Despite the vaunted security fence, the monument was covered in graffiti once again in March 1905. Colonel Edwards reacted with a thundering letter to *The Star*:

As I am returning to India in a few days, I went yesterday afternoon to look at the monument near the observatory, erected to the memory of officers and others of the Indian Army who died during the late war. I feel sure your readers will be sorry to know that the barbed wire fence round it has been broken down, and disgusted to hear that certain individuals have scratched or written their names on the marble tablets ... I trust those responsible for the care of the monument will repair the fence and thus prevent any further desecration.[119]

In later years, the panels were even more badly mutilated. By 1960 vandals had removed most of the lead filling from the letters, and worse followed when some of the original marble tablets were smashed in the late 1980s. The panels were replaced by the War Graves and Graves of Conflict Division of the National Monuments Counci [now known as the South African Heritage Resources Agency], the body which, since the 1960s, has been responsible for maintaining the memorial. Of the original Urdu, Hindi and English inscriptions, only the English ones are left.[120]

HOUSE AT THE CORNER OF SHARP AND ALBERT STREETS, BELLEVUE EAST

LEAVING the middle-class comfort of Troyeville behind him, in August 1906 Gandhi moved into a humble four-roomed house in Bellevue East which he shared with the Polaks. All the rooms were small – none was big enough to accommodate two single beds. Apart from two bedrooms (one for Gandhi, the other for the Polaks), there was a kitchen and a sitting room. Millie Polak was unprepared for the stark and spartan conditions:

> The little house to which I was taken was devoid of any pretence of beauty or of the things that I had been accustomed to look upon as necessities. There were no carpets or rugs to cover the bare deal boards of the floor, no curtains to the windows, only some ugly yellow blinds to keep some suggestion of privacy. Of course, there was not a picture on the yellow-washed walls, and only furniture of the simplest was installed in the house ... I said to Mr Gandhi that I wanted some curtains, some floor-covering and a few other things to make the little house 'home'.[121]

Gandhi remained unconvinced of the need for carpets and curtains, but after some persuasion he good-humouredly agreed to let Mrs Polak have her way.

The house, Millie Polak tells us, was in 'a distant suburb' about four miles from town, facing 'a big stretch of kopje leading away to a district that had been named "the Highlands"'. In the early 1900s Bellevue East was indeed a 'distant suburb'; the koppie is the Observatory-Yeoville Ridge; and just over the crest of this ridge is the suburb of Highlands.

Gandhi's residential address appears – under his own name – in the *United Transvaal Directory* for 1908 as corner Sharp and Albert Streets, Bellevue East. Albert Street branches off Sharp Street, so there are only two possible corners on which the house might have stood. A block of flats now stands on one corner and a modern residence on the other.

Gandhi lived in Bellevue East until the assault of February 1908. Mille Polak wrote of this incident:

> It was while we were occupying this little bungalow that Mr. Gandhi's life was attempted by one of his compatriots and he lay ill for a considerable time at the house of some European friends who had gone to his rescue.

> During his absence from the home in the suburbs we left it and took a small house in town. Here Mr. Gandhi came on his recovery. ... Our little house was in a rather cheap neighbourhood, since, apart from the desire for simplicity, all the available money was used to assist the struggle; and we, therefore, had to take a house at a low rental. The one we occupied was the best we could find at the time, but it was a miserable sort of a place, built in a rather primitive manner.[122]

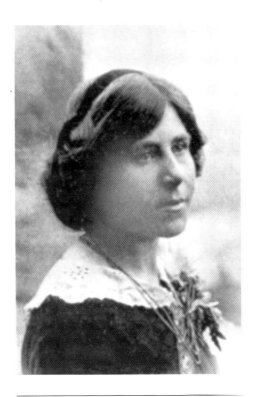

Millie Polak

AFTER BELLEVUE EAST

MILLIE POLAK found one of Gandhi's homes – a house in town which remains unidentified – a wretched place:

My husband, Gandhiji and I, with my baby, had a miserable little house in a fairly busy part of Johannesburg. We could not afford a better one. Money for my family life was very scarce and we had to be near the centre of the struggle. In his [Gandhi's] house there was no proper plumbing, and a makeshift bathroom had been fixed by previous tenants under the stairs; the waste water from the bath ran down the wall outside into a kind of gutter, which ran along a dark passage, and thus the walls were always damp. These conditions helped to produce big slimy slugs that got into the house.[123]

THE KRAAL
15 Pine Road, Orchards.

KALLENBACH'S house in Pine Road, designed by Kallenbach and Reynold, was called The Kraal because of the use of traditional African elements in a European dwelling. The building plans were approved on 28 June 1907.

On the back of a photograph of the house, Kallenbach wrote (in German):

The Kraal, our first house, where Gandhi lived with me for several years. In this house the Rev. J. Doke came many times while writing the book about Gandhi 'An Indian patriot'. 18 Sept. 1928. H. K.

In his biography of Gandhi Doke stated:

I write this in the house in which he usually lives when in Johannesburg. Yonder is the open stoep – there is the rolled-up mattress on which he sleeps.[124]

Gandhi moved in with Kallenbach soon after his recovery. Writing to his brother on 10 June, Kallenbach described three months of life at The Kraal with Gandhi, suggesting that they had been living together in the house since March 1908. In 1937 Kallenbach recalled:

Though we worked in our own offices, we lived in the same rooms – almost in the same bed – and whilst he cooked for us I did the cleaning. I had to account to him for every little item of expenditure …[125]

After Kallenbach's death in 1945, colourful myths arose about Gandhi's stay at The Kraal. Some apocryphal tales appeared in Percy Baneshik's column in *The Star* during the late 1970s and early 1980s.[126] Baneshik points out an intriguing reference to Gandhi in Dennis Wheatley's novel *The Fabulous Valley*, an adventure story published in 1958. The leading character goes to a 'little house in Orchards' where he is told Gandhi once lived and 'used to sleep up there with his goat'. Gandhi did not, in fact, start taking goat's milk until ten years after he left South Africa.

Wheatley reputedly visited The Kraal in about 1949. When Baneshik visited some years later, he was told by his hosts that the house had been 'a refuge for Gandhi when he was on the run from the police'. In reality, far from evading the police, Gandhi often deliberately courted arrest. Baneshik was shown Gandhi's supposed hiding place – a loft under the

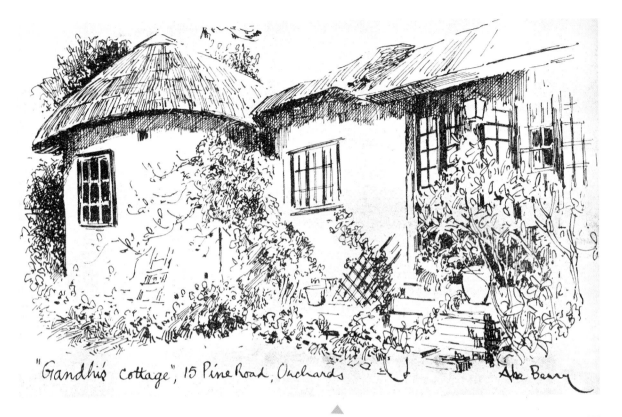

"Gandhi's cottage", 15 Pine Road, Orchards

Abe Berry

Gandhi's cottage in Orchards

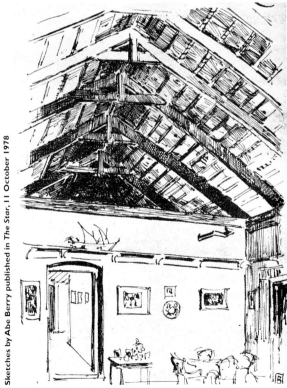

Sketches by Abe Berry published in *The Star*, 11 October 1978

The loft and ladder bracket

thatched roof of the living room, accessible only by ladder. The ladder was gone, although the bracket that had supported it remained. Baneshik reports that the ladder was purchased in about 1950 by some Indians who had removed it for 'most reverent' preservation.

It is not clear whether the ladder was sold or donated. The Transvaal Indian Congress, then the mouthpiece of the Indian community, was approached about the ladder by the occupants of the Kraal. 'We don t have any use for the ladder, so would you please remove it,' said the couple. The Congress treasurer, Jasmat Nanabhai, together with Chotu Makkan and other Congress members fetched the ladder which was later shipped to India and deposited at the Gandhi Memorial Museum in New Delhi.[127] .

MOUNTAIN VIEW AND FAIRWOOD

KALLENBACH and Gandhi lived together for five years, from 1908 to 1913, first at The Kraal, later under canvas at 'The Tents', and finally at Tolstoy Farm. They parted for a brief while in mid-1909 when Gandhi left for London and Kallenbach set up camp at the foot of Linksfield Ridge. After returning from London in December 1909, Gandhi joined Kallenbach at his encampment in Mountain View – a small suburb consisting of five or six streets – where he remained until Tolstoy Farm opened in June 1910.

In true pioneering fashion, Kallenbach opened up and developed virgin land:

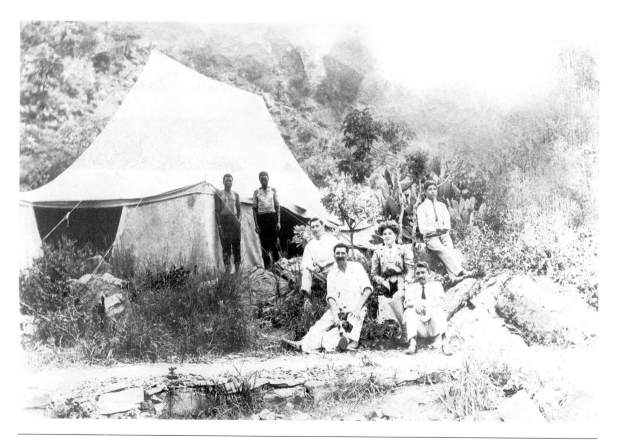

Kallenbach's tent near Mountain View. Gandhi is seated next to Kallenbach, his son Manilal behind him

I lived at Mountain View about one year, from June 1909 to June 1910. I lived there in a tent … [Two bell tents] were occupied by 12 boys and a Boer, who was very proficient in building dry stone walling work. We all made Mountain View in one year what it is today. At first, it was not accessible at all. I was the first purchaser to buy ground against this hill. The ground does not go right up to the top. After the development of the ground, a number of people acquired ground in a similar position. The place is full with indigenous trees, and this is, I think, almost the only hill near Johannesburg on which there are still some left … There is hardly any other place so near Johannesburg where one can roam about half dressed and enjoy one's full liberty and not be troubled so much by outside affairs and persons, as at The Tents.[128]

Kallenbach continued to acquire land around Mountain View after he and Gandhi left for Tolstoy Farm in mid-1910 despite Gandhi's feeling, expressed in a letter in April 1911, that 'I should be far more satisfied with your dispositions if Mountain View could be sold'. Though this wish was to be reiterated in other letters, by January 1913 Kallenbach owned three acres in the area,[129] but he reduced these to a smaller plot in March, probably to meet his debts.[130]

In 1913-1914, while visiting Johannesburg, Gandhi stayed with Kallenbach in Grove Road, which runs through both Mountain View and Fairwood, a tiny adjoining suburb consisting of only 141 stands. Fairwood is enveloped by the more prominent suburbs of Orange Grove and Linksfield. Here, near the foot of the ridge, Kallenbach once more played host to Gandhi.

Kallenbach recorded the visit in his diary:

On the way to Johannesburg Mr. Gandhi, who came from Durban, joined me and together we travelled to Johannesburg. As usual we lived together in my little house in Mountain View, where during my absence a son of his [Manilal] kept house. He had come to my place on 26.8 from Phoenix.[131]

A terse entry in the 1913 *Donaldson and Braby's Transvaal and Rhodesia Directory* reads: Kallenbach, H., architect, Orange Grove. The *United Transvaal Directory* of 1914 provides the following entry: Kallenbach, H., architect, 74-77 Sacke's Bldgs., Joubert St., box 2493, phone 1497. Sts.31-33, Mountain View. The 1915 edition gives as his residence: Stds. 30-32 Grove Road, Mountain View.

In fact, Stands 30-33 are in Fairwood, not Mountain View. There is no record of houses being erected on these stands before the 1930s. According to the available plans for Stand 30, the house was first built in 1933. In the case of stands 31, 32 and 33, the houses date from 1984, 1934 and 1937 respectively. There is however a possibility that other houses could have been erected prior to those dates, as houses were constructed in the vicinity from 1909 onwards.

On 29 August 1913 Kallenbach mentions that he left by tram for Mountain View. By this time tram lines certainly reached as far as Fairwood. As early as 4 October 1904 an advertisement in *The Star* for stands in Fairwood announced: Authorised ELECTRIC TRAMS will run within 500 yards of FAIRWOOD. A similar advertisement in an issue of *The Star* in November 1905 promised: Tram service absolutely assured.

Local tradition has it that Gandhi stayed at 34 Grove Road, on the border of Fairwood and Mountain View. According to one of Percy Baneshik's informants, Gandhi lived at 34 Grove Road, Linksfield Ridge, 'just behind the old Orange Grove Hotel'.[132] However, the house at Number 34 was built for Alexander King Cowie on Stands 27 and 28 in 1909, and Cowie owned the property from 1909 until 1918. Thus it seems Kallenbach was not the owner during the Gandhi period.

Another local legend is that Gandhi hid in a nearby cave on the ridge and that Indian pilgrims visited the cave as late as the 1950s, and eventually the police had it sealed up. Undeveloped veld surrounded the area of the alleged cave, and Gandhi may have gone there in search of solitude or for some other reason.

There is no evidence that he ever evaded arrest, whether by taking refuge in an attic in Orchards or by hiding out in the cave on the hillside in Fairwood. Satyagrahis were duty-bound to suffer the penalties for violating unjust and immoral laws. Leading by example, Gandhi submitted himself willingly to the consequences of disobedience, stoically (even cheerfully) accepting the hardships and discipline of jail.

Johannesburg retains one permanent link with Hermann Kallenbach in Kallenbach Drive which runs through Linksfield. Kallenbach built a house for himself on Linksfield Ridge in 1929 and was living there at the time of his death. Sylvia Pass, the steep, winding road connecting Linksfield and Orange Grove, was the road to his house on the ridge. A great believer in manual labour, Kallenbach insisted on building the road himself, with the help of some black workers. [133] He wanted to name a road on Linksfield Ridge after Gandhi, but the city council refused to accept a 'non-white' name, so he named it Hannaben Street after his niece Hana Lazar.

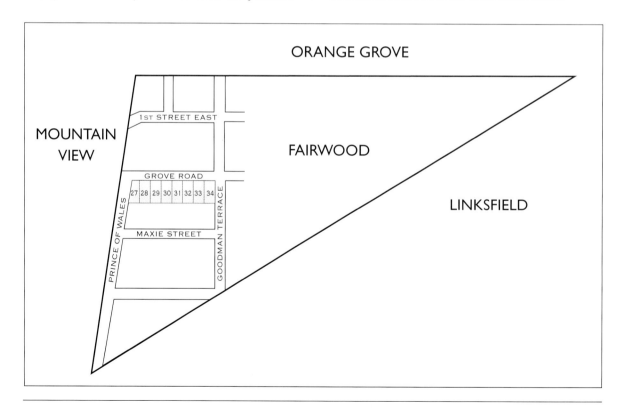

Map of Fairwood showing stands 27-34 on Grove Road

TOLSTOY
FARM

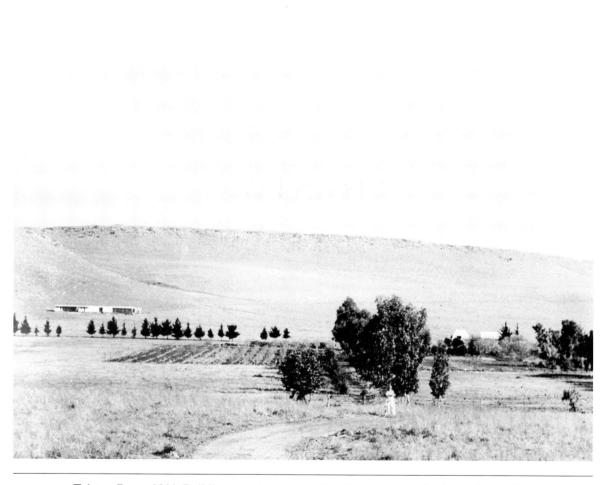

Tolstoy Farm, 1911. Buildings can be seen in the distance near the foot of the ridge

A GRANITE plaque erected by the Gandhi Centenary
Council in 1998 greets visitors near the entrance to
the ruined farmhouse on Tolstoy Farm. It reads:

TOLSTOY FARM

*'The weak became strong on Tolstoy Farm
and labour proved a tonic for all'*

*Tolstoy Farm was originally conceived by M.K. Gandhi as a focal settlement
for Satyagrahis (passive resisters) and the maintenance of their families. This
co-operative commonwealth was an experiment in living together, drawing
families of Satyagrahis closer, in pursuit of a new and simple life, bridging divides
of language, religion, customs, gender and class; and forging values of moral
character, self-reliance, mutual respect, perseverance, tolerance and healthy
organic living. The egalitarian social setting exemplified the inner core of a
Satyagraha struggle, a fight on behalf of truth.*

*Hermann Kallenbach, an architect of German descent living in
Johannesburg, bought 1 100 acres here and gave the use of it to Satyagrahis free
of rent or charge, on May 30 1910. Tolstoy Farm was home to an eclectic group
of some eighty people of diverse cultural, social and religious backgrounds.*

*On the farm there were nearly one thousand fruit bearing trees and a house.
Water was supplied from two wells and a spring. Using their own hands they
built two dormitory blocks, a school house and a workshop for carpentry,
shoemaking, etc. and a kitchen. The structures were all of corrugated iron and
timber.*

The farm was wound down after the great Satyagraha of 1913*.

*Tolstoy Farm was rededicated on May 30 1997 in deep respect for the
men, women and children who under the leadership of Mahatma Gandhi and
the Satyagraha movement strove to make our world a better place for all
humanity and inspire us on this day to build upon their self-less foundation.*

*This statement is innacurate. All the Indians and Kallenbach had left the farm before the great Satyagraha.

TOLSTOY FARM
35 kilometres south-west of Johannesburg and
2 kilometres from Lawley Station

TOLSTOY FARM became the nucleus of the Satyagraha movement during the final phase of the struggle. 'The training imparted at Tolstoy Farm,' wrote Gandhi in 1914, 'proved to be of great use in this last fight'.[134] In his later recollections, he again emphasised the farm's crucial contribution to passive resistance:

I have serious doubts as to whether the struggle could have been prosecuted for eight years, whether we could have secured larger funds, and whether the thousands of men who participated in the last phase of the struggle would have borne their share of it, if there had been no Tolstoy Farm.[135]

After returning from London in 1909, Gandhi saw the need for a resistance base near Johannesburg where Satyagrahis and their families could be sustained. Poor Indians in and around Johannesburg were the mainstay of the movement. When breadwinners were imprisoned or unemployed as a result of political activism, their families depended on cash handouts from the Passive Resistance Council. What was needed, Gandhi reasoned, was a self-supporting co-operative commonwealth, after the pattern of the Phoenix settlement he had established near Durban in 1904. A Transvaal settlement would save money, boost morale, and help co-ordinate their activities.[136]

The generosity of Hermann Kallenbach helped convert Gandhi's idea into reality. Kallenbach bought a farm at Lawley and on 30 May 1910 placed it at the disposal of the Satyagrahis, rent free, for as long as their campaign lasted.

It was Kallenbach who named the farm after Leo Tolstoy, the Russian author who gave up his wealth and took to a life of poverty and labour. As Gandhi explained to Tolstoy:

No writings have so deeply touched Mr Kallenbach as yours; and, as a spur to further effort in living up to the ideals held before the world by you, he has taken the liberty, after consultation with me, of naming his farm after you.[137]

Gandhi, too, was a great admirer of the Russian, and began corresponding with him in October 1909. The Indian leader's ideals, practised at Tolstoy Farm, of material simplicity, self-discipline and manual labour, were akin to those taught by Tolstoy.

The farm, which covered 1 100 acres, was two miles long and three-quarters of a mile broad. About 1 000 fruit-bearing trees – including apricots, peaches, oranges, plums, figs and almonds – already grew there. Water was supplied by two wells and a small spring, and the soil was fertile.[138]

The original buildings consisted of a shed and a small, dilapidated house which had been built by the previous owner at the foot of a hill. With self-help their watchword from the outset, the Satyagrahis built accommodation for themselves. The initial work was done by six Indians and Kallenbach, who all lived together in the original house. Soon the number of settlers increased, and after two months of living in tents, they were all housed in new structures of iron and wood.

Six weeks after moving onto the farm. Gandhi and Kallenbach with a group of settlers. Behind them is the original farmhouse, a small corrugated iron building with a porch on only one side.

Satyagrahis did much of the unskilled construction work, with some help from African labourers. Naturally Kallenbach was the architect, and he also paid the building costs, which amounted to £600. Stonework for the foundations was done by a white mason. Suitable stones were available on the farm, but had to be rolled quite a distance to the building site. Indian carpenters, including Narandas Damania, offered their services. Timber, wrote Gandhi, was plentiful at the site:

> The timber too could be had ready-made in all sizes required. All we had to do was to cut it to measure. There were not many doors or windows to be prepared. Hence it was that quite a number of buildings could be erected within such a short space of time.[139]

Within six months of starting the settlement, the residents completed three large corrugated iron sheds,

two of them 53 feet long and the third 77 feet. One of these served as the women's dormitory. The men's quarters were erected some distance away, forming a separate block complete with laundry and kitchen facilities.[140] Accommodation was provided for ten women and sixty men. A third building was a combination of offices, a school, and a workshop for carpentry and sandal-making.

The common misapprehension that Kallenbach occupied a free-standing house at Tolstoy Farm stems from a line in *Satyagraha in South Africa* in which Gandhi writes 'we had to erect a house for Kallenbach'. But Gandhi's sentence continues '… and by its side a school house, as well as a workshop for carpentry, shoemaking, etc.'[141] Far from occupying a separate house, Kallenbach had a room at one end of a long shed, with a verandah between it and the schoolroom. Time and again Gandhi refers to Kallenbach's 'room'. Writing to Kallenbach on 27 August 1911 regarding a patient coming to the

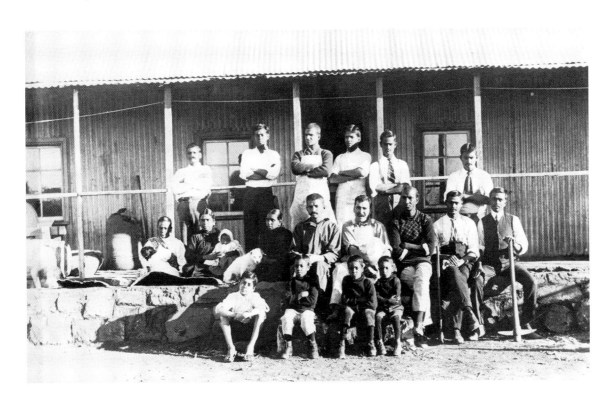

farm, Gandhi noted: 'I propose to use your room for him'. He reported on 16 September 1911 that the floor had been re-laid: 'the verandah between your room and the school will be finished by the end of the week'. And concerning G K Gokhale's visit to the farm in November 1912, Gandhi stated: 'He [Gokhale] had been up in Mr Kallenbach's room'. [142]

Distanced as it was from the distractions of urban life, Tolstoy Farm provided opportunities for simple living in harmony with nature. This was ideal for Gandhi, who organised the farm as an experiment in community living. Daily life was characterised by co-operation, hard work and voluntary poverty. There were no beds and little other furniture – residents slept on the floor. Both adults and children grew their own vegetables and fruit. The diet was vegetarian and smoking and drinking were prohibited.

At its height Tolstoy Farm supported a community of about fifty adults and thirty children but by April 1912 most of the Satyagrahis' families had left, since passive resistance had been suspended after an interim agreement with Smuts. Gandhi left the farm on 9 January 1913, leaving behind only Kallenbach and the Africans who lived there.

Kallenbach rented out the farm from February 1913, reserving fifty acres, including the three large sheds, in case they were needed again by passive resisters. He transferred the property to W H Humphries under Deed of Transfer 14040/34 and Humphries later transferred the farm to Anglovaal Brick and Tile Company under Deed of Transfer 14041/34. Tolstoy Farm gradually faded from the collective consciousness of the Indian community.

Efforts to revive public interest in the farm began in the late 1960s when the Transvaal Gandhi Centenary Council (TGCC), established to mark the centenary of Gandhi's birth (1969), conceived the idea of preserving it as a monument. After negotiations, the company donated a small portion of the farm – a brick house and four acres of surrounding land – to the TGCC in 1974. The house, which was very run down, was assumed to be Kallenbach's original dwelling. There was no sign of other buildings on the site.

The house was restored by the Centenary Council in about 1982 but by 1996 the building had been almost completely destroyed by vandals, leaving only stumps of walls. After consultation and soul searching, the TGCC resolved to restore the house only up to plinth level and to cement the floor. This is the way it has remained – only the floor space of the original house can be seen.

The vandalised building attracted much attention, but it is doubtful whether Kallenbach ever occupied it, though he might have built it in the 1920s to attract tenants. Early photographs show that the Satyagrahis built closer to the southern ridge, some distance from the spot occupied by the plinth structure.

The only traces of the Satyagrahis which have survived on Tolstoy Farm are a scattering of fruit trees here and there which recall the flourishing orchards which they pruned and tended. Peppercorn trees planted almost ninety years ago surround an outdoor auditorium built by the Centenary Council in the 1980s.

But, though the man-made structures associated with Gandhi may have disappeared, the flora, the peaceful surroundings and the largely unspoilt natural environment still provide a physical link with his original community.

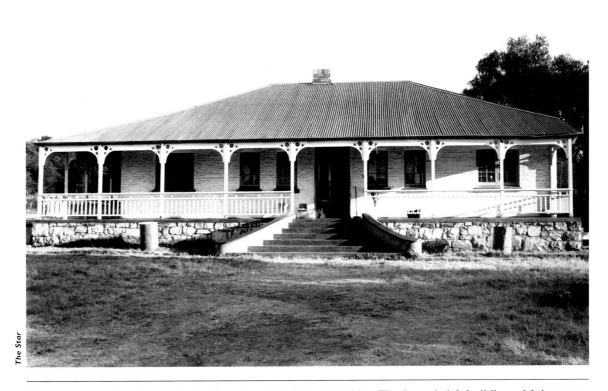

The renovated farmhouse, built after Gandhi left South Africa. The large brick building with its wrap-around veranda is strikingly different from the original house

APPENDIX

Speech by High Commissioner Gopalkrishna Gandhi
at the rededication of Valliamma's grave
20 April 1997

THERE IS something wisp-like about you, Valliamma, that eludes us. No longer a child, not yet a woman, what made you decide to join the marchers, to become a revolutionary? The others were all much older, were they not? Mostly married women and men stung into action by the law that disrecognised Indian marriages. You were barely seventeen and unmarried.

You joined them, nevertheless. Joined them on the long dusty march, down the fields, down the roads, eating little, sleeping less, you joined them. I can picture you, jumping over the runnels of water, doe-stepped, with the light of youth in your eyes, helping the older marchers along. I can imagine you comforting the mother who lost her babe in the gushing stream, can see you being the life of the determined group of marchers, the Transvaal party . Did they sing as they marched, Tamil songs, perhaps with ones in Hindi or in Gandhibhai's language, Gujarati? I wonder what your thoughts were during the march? You had not been to India (as far as we know) so you could not have pictured your ancestral village, its little temple, its paddy fields.

You were South African, of South African earth, knowing only its sugar cane acres and its mines. But whatever your thoughts were, they were certainly about life, about living, about the future. Death could not have entered your mind. Certainly not your impending death.

You were there when the police arrived, raising, I imagine, a mushroom of arrogant dust. You were there when the arrests began. I wonder what you felt when you entered the prison gates, when the iron doors clanged shut behind you. You, a child of the sun and the air, what did your mind say when you entered the dark and the damp of Maritzburg jail? Did Kasturba speak to you about what lay ahead, did someone say to you Child, so this is it! We have chosen to suffer so here we are … ?

But perhaps it was you Valliamma … yes it must have been you who took the others' trembling hands into your own and raised their morale, in whatever language that came to you. You do not need to know another's language, do you, to comfort her or him. You only need human care and will.

That, Valliamma, you certainly had. You had will. The will to dare, to die.

When you took ill, Valliamma, did you … fear the worst? Did any doctor come; perhaps some indifferent doctor did come but you did not like to be examined by some strange man who seemed not too keen to examine you. On the other hand, he perhaps was a caring soul and I do him injustice. You must understand, Valliamma, that I and all those present here are so conscious of the venality of the system that jailed you that despite ourselves we monsterise the whole scene. Perhaps it was not a man but a woman doctor who saw in you one like herself but also a very different person - supremely different, radiant, confident. On the other hand, Valliamma, perhaps no doctor came at all … Professor Nicky Padayachee, a doctor who now works at the Johannesburg City Council as Chief Executive Officer, is determined to get to the exact circumstances of your illness.

The fact remains, Valliamma, that when you left the jail, you were grievously ill. The food you and the other women marchers from in the Natal party and from the Transvaal party like yourself had been given was unfit for consumption. And you will remember you were given hard labour. You had been assigned to do laundry work. To have to live on food that was virtually inedible and then to wash clothes … That must have been hard. You had traipsed through the march, entered the jail-cage at Maritzburg like a bird. But by the time the prison gates opened, ever so creakily, ever so grudgingly, to let you return home, you were too ill - and here again I am imagining the scene – too ill to walk. You must have been helped out by the other women Satyagrahis. Paavam, kuzhanthai … they must have said, poor child … Did you hush their words of concern, Valliamma with your special confidence: ' … Naan paavamum ille, kuzhanthaiyum ille …' ('I am neither poor nor am I a child').

The Mahatma visited you when you were ill. The Mahatma …, who is that? You ask.

I should have known better; you did not know him by that name. Gandhibhai, as he was known to you and your generation here, came to be called Mahatma in India, some years later, Valliamma. You

were very ill indeed when he saw you. Your emaciated body was a terrible thing, he said, to behold. When he asked if you did not repent of your having gone to jail, you said to him: 'Repent? I am even now ready to go to jail again if I am arrested …' He persisted with his quiet questioning, Valliamma.

'But what if it results in your death?' he asked. Now, ordinarily, people visiting those who are unwell do not talk about death, even though the possibility of the patient's death is uppermost in their minds. But Gandhi was not an ordinary sort of man, you see. He too was utterly unafraid. You were speaking as one Satyagrahi to another.

'I do not mind it, you told him. Who would not love to die for one's motherland?'

Motherland … Again, Valliamma, I wonder if you spoke in Tamil. Perhaps you did and there was an interpreter. Perhaps you said Thainaadu … Perhaps, Naadu or Desam. You meant your ancestral home, the village you had heard of, your province, your mother India; but you also meant the cause of Indian self-respect in South Africa … And somewhere in the distant horizon, the cause of human self-respect and dignity in the whole of South Africa.

We can tell you now, Valliamma, that this year when we are gathered at your gravesite is the fiftieth year of India's freedom. We became free fifty years ago under the same leader who led your pilgrim band here. He returned to India the year after he visited you, the year after your great march, the year after your martyrdom. He returned a hero, Valliamma. A hero who had succeeded here, who had brought the white government of South Africa to agree to an honourable redressal of the grievances.

But his success was enabled in no small measure by that great march, Valliamma, by the jailings, the sufferings of those pilgrims - prisoners so uniquely symbolised by your martyrdom. 'The name Valliamma will live,' he later wrote, 'as long as India lives'.

He has not given such praise to many.

Valliamma, where you lie is a headstone that was unveiled in his presence. It is in fact a milestone, a great and unique landmark in the history of India's freedom from colonialism and the liberation of South Africa from apartheid. For South Africa too is now free. Its President Nelson Mandela has said on many an occasion that what Gandhi did in South Africa inspired the sons and daughters of this country to organise themselves in a mass struggle to fight for their own freedom.

This, your grave, which had slipped out of public memory for years under apartheid, was re-discovered thanks to the great efforts of Professor James Hunt and the never-say-die perseverence of persons like Enuga Reddy and Ramy Pillay. You do not know their names, Valliamma. But your name is a legend with them, with all of us. Your grave is not a grave as much as it is a cradle of the revolution that won its goal here and then went on to win it in India too. Valliamma, you will be pleased to learn that Nagappen, who died in 1909 and of who you must have heard, has also had his grave re-discovered here, not far from yours. Thanks to the authorities here and of people like Mr Alan Buff who has re-accessioned old cemetery records, Nagappen too is being comemorated here. Another Satyagrahi, another Tamil, another Indian, another South African, another martyr. Your family is present here, Valliamma, your brothers and sisters are here. And the honours are being done here today by the veteran South African leader, Walter Sisulu, in the presence of the decendants of Ahmed Mohammed Cachalia and Thambi Naidoo, E I Asvat, L W Ritch and Nana Sita - all of whom were Gandhi's associates or followers here. In other words, *your* family is here together with your extended family. The Chief Minister of Tamil Nadu, Kalaignar M Karunanidhi has sent a special message for this occasion, which will be read in a moment. He has also suggested that a couplet from the great Thirukkural be inscribed on the site. It is a moving couplet that says it all.

I am reminded particularly today of one person who was with you in the Maritzburg jail: Kasturba. Both of you were prisoners together and she too became a martyr. Coincidentally, she was to die on the very same date, February 22, exactly thirty years later, in 1944. Both of you are Maritzburg co-prisoners and your deaths are not deaths, but proclamations of the indomitable spirit of Satyagraha.

So, wisp-like and elusive as you are, Valliamma, your martyrdom is a monument to freedom. You died so that your compatriots could live in freedom. But Valliamma, I would be false to your memory if I did not say that the freedom we have achieved in India is still incomplete in many ways. But in one respect more than any other. Our women, Valliamma, are not half as free as they should be. The majority of our women are not yet regarded by the majority of our men as their equal partners; they are not yet empowered. Empowered is not a word that was used in your days; it is a relatively new word. But you symbolised empowerment. The majority of our women are expected generally within the first twenty years of their lives, to be daughters, sisters, daughters-in-law, wives, mothers. That is, to be everything but themselves.

Only a small proportion of them are in the professions, an even smaller in our legislatures and parliament. But more importantly, their absolute numbers in India demand attention. For every 1 000 males there are not 1 000 females as there ought to be but only 930. Why? Is it that Indian women cannot access health care in the same way as Indian men can? Is it that the girl child, the girl infant and the female foetus face discrimination? It is a fact, Valliamma, that Indian women, particularly in rural and tribal India, have to walk several kilometres –

not two or three but ten, twenty or thirty, every day to fetch water and fuel wood. It is known that very often the head load of fuel is heavier than the girl or woman who is carrying it. Ours is a very unequal society, Valliamma. It is patriarchal, to put it gently. It is crudely male-dominated, to put it more directly. Had you been alive, I know that you would have fought to change this.

The situation is changing, but not fast enough. In a recently inaugurated programme a pioneering scheme for female literacy has been announced. It is going to benefit women in states where female literacy rates are very low. Your province, Tamil Nadu, has already shown how change can be brought about. In the district of Pudukkottai, women have thought of a novel way of reaching unaccessed villages to spread female literacy. A pioneering District Collector, a woman by the name of Sheela Rani Chunkath, encouraged women literacy workers to take to the bicycle and move in large numbers of cycles to these villages. A bicycle revolution started in that district with tens and hundreds of women beginning a kind of movement on bicycles, spreading the message not just of female literacy but of female *mobility, of momentum and progress*. Songs were composed bringing to the cycle revolution a new spirit of freedom and adventure. How marvellously, Valliamma, would *you* have led this revolution!

In a poem to Gandhi after his assassination the poetess Sarojini Naidu said to him

'Rest NOT in Peace!' You, Valliamma, have rested in a kind of artificial peace all these decades since 1914. Now, bestir yourself. And rest not in peace until the freedoms of India and South Africa reach their completion with their daughters leading their sons to equality.

NOTES

GANDHI IN TOWN

1   Mohandas Karamchand Gandhi, *Gandhi's Autobiography,* Washington 1948, pp 145-6.

2   *The Transvaal Critic* of 11 March 1898 reported on the splendid hydraulic lift at Permanent Buildings. There has been some controversy about whether this was the first lift installed in Johannesburg. *The Star* of 21 September 1936 conferred this distinction on a lift installed in Frazer Street in August 1897 for the Transvaal and Delagoa Bay Collieries Co.

3   *Cape Argus*, 25 April 1983.

4   Mrs Carrie Chapman Catt, 'Gandhi in South Africa'. In *The Woman Citizen*, March 1922. Reproduced in Blanche Watson, *Gandhi and Non-violent Resistance, The Non-Co-operation Movement in India: Gleanings from the American Press*. Madras 1923.

5   Albert West's reminiscences appear in the *Illustrated Weekly of India*, Bombay, 3-31 October 1965.

6   *Autobiography*, p 326.

7   *Longlands Transvaal Directory*, 1906.

8   Autobiography, p 326.

9   Ibid, p 328.

10 *Cape Argus*, 25 April 1983.

11 *The Star* of 14 July 1914 stated that at the time of Gandhi's final departure from Johannesburg in June 1914 he was living temporarily in Anderson Street. It is possible that Gandhi had returned to his old room. However, it is more likely that he was staying at or near 15 Anderson Street, where he had set up a temporary office in January 1914. (Mohandas Karamchand Gandhi, *The Collected Works of Mahatma Gandhi*, Delhi 1958, Vol XII, p 664). 15 Anderson Street is far to the west of the Court Chambers site.

12 Chandrashanker Shukla (ed), *Incidents of Gandhiji s life*, Bombay 1949, p 232.

13 Joseph J Doke, *M K Gandhi*, Delhi 1967, p 10.

14 Autobiography, p 348.

15 G A Leyds, *A History of Johannesburg*, Cape Town 1964, p 144.

16 Anna H Smith, *Johannesburg Street Names*, Cape Town 1971, p 551.

17 *Selected works*, Vol. III, p 203.

18 The settlement was short-lived. Smuts did not repeal the Registration Act, and later denied having promised any concessions. Gandhi accused Smuts of reneging on their agreement.

19 William E Cursons, *Joseph Doke*, Johannesburg 1929, p 144.

20 Gerhard-Mark van der Waal, *From Mining Camp to Metropolis*, Pretoria 1987, p 132.

21 *Longlands Transvaal Directory* 1906. Johannesburg, p 259.

22 *Incidents of Gandhiji s life*, p 228.

23 The discrepancy in the street numbers can be traced to the 1940s when the numbering was changed by the City Council.

24 Autobiography, p 322.

25 Margaret Chatterjee, *Gandhi and his Jewish Friends*, Basingstoke 1992, p 172.

26 *Indian Opinion*, 5 March 1910.

27 *Collected works*, Vol. XI, p 344.

28 *The Star*, 14 July 1914; *Rand Daily Mail*, 27 April 1983.

29 Souvenir of the Passive Resistance Movement in South Africa, 1906-1914, p 10.

30 *The Star*, 10 March 1905.

31 *Collected works*, Vol. XII, p 171.

32 A footnote in Vol XII of Gandhi's *Collected Works* mistakenly states that the memorial service for Doke was held at the Grahamstown Baptist Church, Johannesburg, of which he was pastor (p 175). Doke served as minister of the Grahams-

town Baptist Church in the Eastern Cape from 1903 until he moved to Johannesburg in 1907.

33 *Collected works*, Vol. XII, p 176.

BRAAMFONTEIN AND HOSPITAL HILL

34 Anna H Smith, *Johannesburg Street Names*, Cape Town 1971, p220.

35 *Rand Daily Mail*, 11 February 1908.

36 William E Cursons. Joseph Doke. Johannesburg 1929, p 144.

37 Mohandas Karamchand Gandhi, *The Selected Works of Mahatma Gandhi* Vol III, p229.

38 James D Hunt, *Gandhi and the Nonconformists*, New Delhi c1986, p 100.

39 *Incidents of Gahdhiji's Life*, Bombay 1949, p40.

40 Ibid.

41 Rose Norwich, Synagogues on the Witwatersrand and Pretoria Before 1932, Master of Architecture dissertation, University of the Witwatersrand 1988, Vol I, p 151.

42 *South African Gandhi*, pp 600-604.

43 Submission to the National Monuments Council on the 'Native Gaol', the Fort, Hospital Hill, Johannesburg: 1995-02-15. Compiled by M Birch and submitted by M Martinson.

44 Flo Bird, *The Old Fort, Johannesburg*, Submission to the Parliamentary Portfolio Committee of Arts, Culture, Language, Science and Technology by F Bird on 6 June 1996.

45 *South African Gandhi*, p 581.

46 He went to India via London.

47 *Collected Works*, Vol XII, pp 486-7.

48 *The Star*, 21 April 1997.

49 David Y Saks, 'Right-hand Man of the Mahatma: Hermann Kallenbach, Gandhi and Satyagraha'. In *Jewish Affairs*, Autumn 1998.

50 As observed by Professor J D Hunt in July 1997. The inscription above this is in Tamil and below it in Gujarati.

51 Interview with Alan Buff of the Johannesburg Cemeteries Department.

52 In his article *In the Footsteps of Mahatma Gandhi*, Homer Jack describes the Valliamma headstone as 'crumbling'. The memorial could not, however, have been disintegrating when he visited the site in 1952. Jack may have been misled by the fading light of dusk for, by his own account, the 'deepening shadows of tall eucalyptus trees' already covered the cemetery.

53 The inscription above this is in Tamil and below it in Gujurati.

54 *Souvenir of the Passive Resistance Movement in South Africa, 1906-1914*, p 25

55 *Indian Opinion*, 5 August 1914, reporting Gandhi's speech to the Johannesburg Tamil community on 15 July 1914.

WESTERN DISTRICTS

56 Arnold Benjamin, *Lost Johannesburg*, p 32.

57 *Rand Daily Mail*, 12 September 1906.

58 *South African Gandhi*, p 298.

59 Incidents of Gandhiji s life, p 242.

60 *Collected works*, Vol. IV, p 406.

61 *The Star*, 7 June 1983.

62 *Collected Works* Vol VI, pp 394-408, p510.

63 Ibid, Vol XII, p 272.

64 *Transvaal Leader*, 14 July 1914.

65 Narendra Dhirajlal Pandya, *The Samaj*, Johannesburg 1982, pp 14-36.

66 *South African Gandhi*, p 1198.

67 Interview with N G Patel, Chairman of the Gandhi Centenary Council.

68 Melanie Yap, *Colour, Confusion and Concessions*, pp 137-168.

69 Ibid, p 149.

70 *Selected Works*, Vol. III, p 200.

71 Yap, p 232.

72 *Indian Opinion*, 16 September 1905.

73 Yap, p 234.

74 Carrim, p 6.

75 *Illustrated Weekly of India*, October 1965.

76 Joseph J Doke, *M K Gandhi*, Delhi 1967, pp 76-77.

77 Elsabé Brink, *Newtown, Old Town*, Johannesburg 1994, p 12.

78 *Indian Opinion*, 2 April 1904.

79 *Autobiography*, 1948, p 351.

80 *Park Station*. Johannesburg, Transnet Museum, 1992?

81 *Incidents of Gandhiji s Life*, pp. 44-45.

82 *Collected Works*, Vol. IX, p 218.

83 *Indian Opinion*, 4 December 1909.

84 *Incidents of Gandhiji's Life*, p 242.

85 Ebrahim Mahomed Mahida, *History of Muslims in South Africa*. Durban: Arabic Study Circle, 1993, p 49.

86 *Collected Works*, Vol. VIII, p 33.

87 D G Tendulkar, *Mahatma*, Delhi 1960, Vol I, p 95.

88 *Selected Works*, Vol III, p 277.

89 Carrim, pp 6-7.

90 *Indian Opinion*, 6 March 1904.

91 *A Documentary History of Indian South Africans*, p 118.

92 Maureen Swan, *Gandhi*, Johannesburg 1985, p 121.

93 *Collected Works*, Vol V, p 392.

94 *Braby's Commercial Directory*, 1960. Pageview's Avalon should not be confused with the Fordsburg cinema of the same name.

95 Braby's Commercial Directory, 1970; Philip Bawcombes's Johannesburg, p 127.

96 Carrim, p 74.

97 Interview with Mr Abdul Bhamjee.

98 V Luxman, The History of Brixton Cemetery, pp 2-3.

99 *Selected Works*, p 323; Pandya, pp 21-22.

100 Johannesburg Town Council Minutes, Adjourned Ordinary Meeting (272nd), 24 September 1912, p 791.

101 Luxman, p 4.

102 Inscription below in Gujarati.

103 *History of the Southern Transvaal Football Association* ... Compiled and edited by John Sinclair. Johannesburg: The Association, 1983, p. 60.

104 *Collected Works*, Vol XI, p 597, 600.

IN THE SUBURBS

105 Polak, p 19.

106 Ibid, p 18.

107 Judith Watt, The Gandhi House. In *House and Leisure* October 1994.

108 *Sunday Times*, 29 September and 6 October 1996.

109 Hunt, Further notes on the Gandhi house in Troyeville (unpublished), 8 October 1996.

110 *Selected Works*, Vol III, pp132-3.

111 Polak, pp 70-71.

112 Major-General Sir E R P Woodgate (1845-1900) was that relatively rare phenomenon in modern warfare – a general who was killed, or at least, mortally wounded in battle. A veteran of other African campaigns, including the Anglo-Zulu War of 1879, Woodgate was in command of the troops who occupied Spioenkop on the night of 23 January 1900. During the battle the next day, he was struck above the eye by a pellet from a bursting shrapnel shell and died after several agonising weeks. The battle lasted nine days in all, with the British suffering a major defeat. The British suffered about 2 600 casualties, of which about 1900 occurred on 24 January alone. Boer losses totalled less than 200. Woodgate was buried at St John's Church Cemetery, Mooi River.

113 Doke, p 67.

114 *Selected Works*, Vol III, p 106.

115 Johannesburg Town Council Minutes (71st Meeting), 29 October 1902.

116 Wilson, W H *After Pretoria*, Vol 1, pp 256, 404.

117 Records of the Observatory Park Cemetery are kept by the War Graves and Graves of Conflict Division of the South African Heritage Resources Agency (File WG 251).

118 Johannesburg Town Council Minutes (101st Meeting), 16 September 1903.

119 Letter from Colonel A H M Edwards, Commandant of Volunteers, Transvaal, in *The Star*, 27 March 1905.

120 Knox, p 59.

121 Polak, pp 70-72.

122 Ibid, pp 92-95.

123 Millie Graham Polak, My South African Days with Gandhiji. In the *Indian Review*, Madras, October 1964.

124 Doke, p 109.

125 *Harijan*, 29 May 1937.

126 *The Star*, 11 October 1978 and 7 June 1983.

127 Interview with Mr Chotu Makkan, Chairman of the Transvaal Hindu Seva Samaj.

128 Letter to a friend, 17 March 1913.

129 Letter to Isabella Fyvie Mayo, 13 January 1913.

130 Kallenbach records the end of 'Auction sales of Mountain View Stands' on 20 March 1913.

131 Bartolf, p 30.

132 *The Star*, 11 October 1978.

133 *Sunday Times*, 23 March 1945.

TOLSTOY FARM

134 *Collected Works*, Vol XII, p 520.

135 *Selected Works*, Vol III, p 352.

136 Bhana, p 99.

137 Gandhi's letter to Tolstoy dated 15 August 1910.

138 Bartolf, p 21.

139 Selected Works, Vol III, p 324.

140 Bhana, p 95.

141 *Selected Works*, Vol III, p 321

142 Ibid, p 339.

SELECT BIBLIOGRAPHY

Bartolf, Christian and Sarid, Isa. 1997. *Hermann Kallenbach: Mahatma Gandhi's friend in South Africa*. Berlin, Gandhi-Informations-Zentrum.

Bartolf, Christian (ed). 1997. Letter to a Hindoo: Taraknath Das, Leo Tolstoi and Mahatma Gandhi. Berlin: Gandhi Information Centre.

Benjamin, Arnold. *Lost Johannesburg*. 1979. Johannesburg, MacMillan.

Bhana, Surendra. The Tolstoy Farm: Gandhi's Experiment in Co-operative Commonwealth. November 1975. In *South African History Journal 7*.

Bhana, Surendra and Bridglal Pachai (eds). 1984. *A Documentary History Of Indian South Africans*. Cape Town: David Philip.

Bird, Flo. *The Old Fort, Johannesburg: Proposals for the Development of the Buildings and Land of the Fort Site for a Museum of Racial Tolerance and a Centre of Reconciliation*. Submission to the Parliamentary Portfolio Committee of Arts, Culture, Language, Science and Technology by F Bird on 6 June 1996.

Brink, Elsabé. 1994. *Newtown, Old Town*. Johannesburg: MuseuMAfricA, 1994.

Brown, Judith M and Prozesky, Martin (eds). 1996. *Gandhi and South Africa: Principles and Politics* Pietermaritzburg: University of Natal Press.

Carrim, Nazir. 1990. *Fietas: A Social History of Pageview, 1948-1998*. Johannesburg: Save Pageview Association.

Chatterjee, Margaret. 1992. *Gandhi and his Jewish Friends*. Basingstoke: MacMillan.

Cursons, William E. 1929. *Joseph Doke: The Missionary-hearted*. Johannesburg: Christian Literature Depot.

Doke, Joseph J. 1967. *M.K. Gandhi: An Indian Patriot in South Africa*. Delhi: Publications Division.

Gandhi, Mohandas Karamchand. 1958. *The collected works of Mahatma Gandhi*. Delhi, Publications Division.

———— c1948. *Gandhi's Autobiography: The Story of my Experiments With Truth*. Washington: Public Affairs Press.

_____ 1968? *The selected works of Mahatma Gandhi*. Vol. III: *Satyagraha in South Africa*. Ahmedabad: Navajivan.

Reddy, E S and Gandhi, Gopalkrishna (eds). 1993. *Gandhi and South Africa, 1914-1948*. Ahmedabad: Navajivan.

Hunt, James D. c1986. *Gandhi and the Nonconformists: Encounters in South Africa*. New Delhi: Promilla.

Chandrashanker, Shukla (Ed). 1949. *Incidents of Gandhiji's life*. Bombay: Vora.

Jack, Homer A. 1953? In the Footsteps of Mahatma Gandhi. In *Friends Intelligencer*.

Knox, Patricia and Gutsche, Thelma. 1947. *Do you know Johannesburg?* Vereeniging: Unie-Volkspers.

Leyds, G. A. 1964. *A History of Johannesburg: The Early Years*. Cape Town: Nasionale Boekhandel.

Luxman, V. 1995. *The History of Brixton Cemetery*.

Mahida, Ebrahim Mahomed. 1993. *History of Muslims in South Africa*. Durban: Arabic Study Circle.

Meiring, Hannes, van der waal, GM and gritter, Wilhelm. 1986. *Early Johannesburg: Its Buildings and its People*. Cape Town: Human & Rousseau.

Pandya Narendra Dhirajlal. 1982. *The Samaj: An*

Outline History of the Transvaal Hindu Seva Samaj, 1932-1982. Johannesburg: PNJ.

Pillay, Bala. 1976. *British Indians in the Transvaal: Trade, Politics, and Imperial Relations, 1885-1906.* London: Longman.

Polak, Millie Graham. 1931. *Mr. Gandhi: The Man.* London: George Allen & Unwin.

Saks, David Y. Satyagraha: Love in a Firm Cause. In *Vuka,* Vol. 2, No. 3, June-July 1997.

——— 1998. Right-hand man of the Mahatma: Hermann Kallenbach, Gandhi and Satyagraha. In *Jewish Affairs,* Autumn.

Smith, Anna H. *Johannesburg Street Names: A Dictionary of Street, Suburb and Other Place Names Compiled to the End of 1968.* 1971. Cape Town: Juta.

Meer, Fatima (ed). 1996. *The South African Gandhi : An Astract of Speeches and Writings of M.K. Gandhi..* 2nd ed. Durban: Madiba.

Souvenir of the Passive Resistance Movement in South Africa, 1906-1914. 1914. Golden number of *Indian Opinion.*

Swan, Maureen. 1985. *Gandhi : The South African Experience.* Johannesburg: Ravan Press.

Tendulkar, D.G. 1960. *Mahatma: Life of Mohandas Karamchand Gandhi.* Vol. I. Revised edition. Delhi: Publications Division.

Thomson, Mark. 1993. *Gandhi and his Ashrams.* London: Sangam.

Van der Waal, Gerhard-Mark. 1987. *From Mining Camp to Metropolis: The Buildings of Johannesburg, 1886-1940.* Pretoria: Chris van Rensburg.

Watt, Judith. 1994. The Gandhi House. *In House and Leisure,* October.

West, Albert. In the Early Days with Gandhi. In *Illustrated Weekly of India,* Bombay, October 3, 10, 17 and 31.

Wilson, W.H. 1902. *After Pretoria: The Guerilla War.* London: Amalgamated Press.

Yap, Melanie and Man, Dianne Leong. C1996. *Colour, Confusion and Concessions: The History of the Chinese in South Africa.* Hong Kong: Hong Kong University Press.

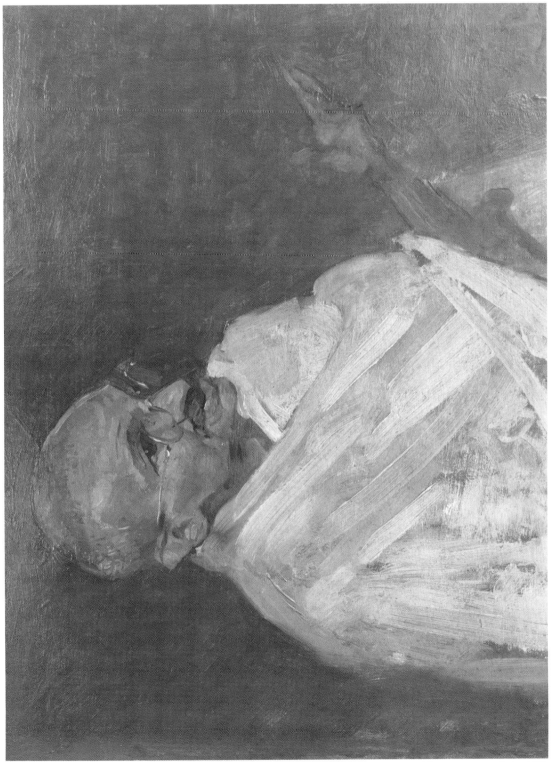

Mahatma Gandhi

A portrait painted from life by J H Amshewitz 1931, MuseuMAfricA

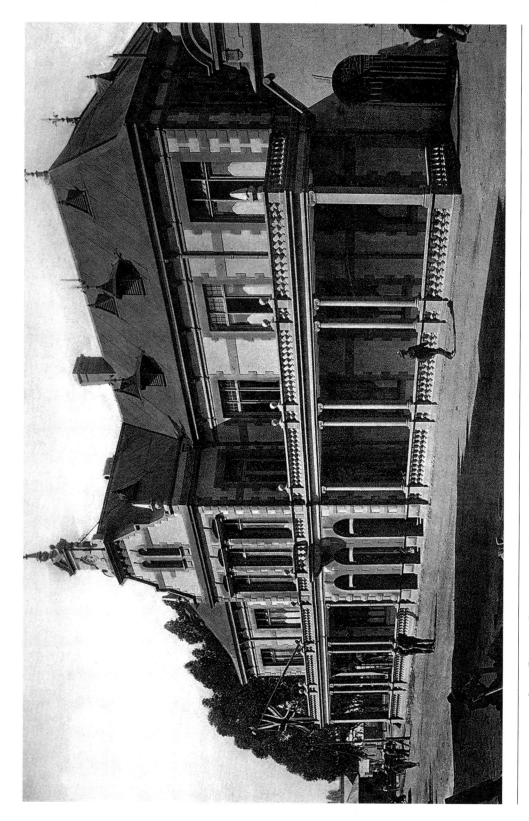

Law Courts, Government Square. Gandhi appeared here as an attorney and as a political offender

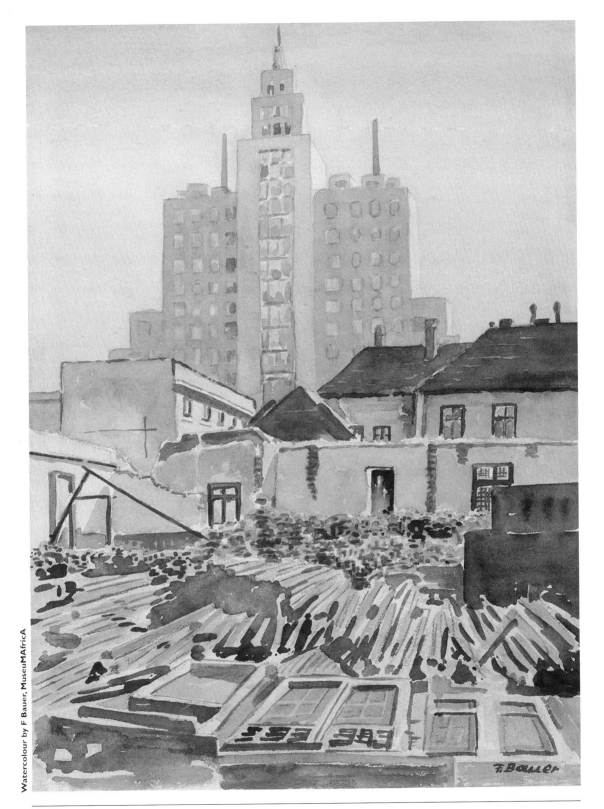

Demolition of the old Law Courts, overlooked by Escom House, 1948

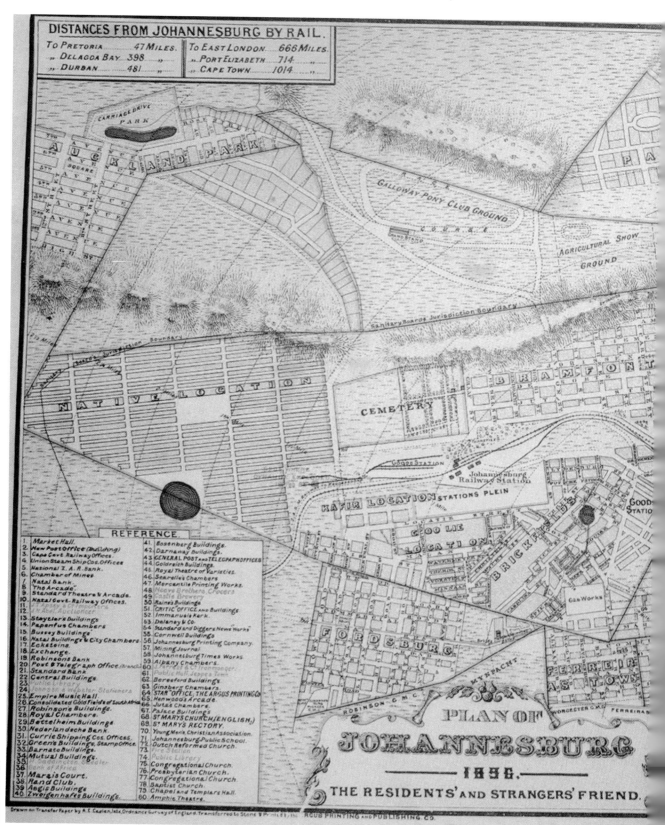

DISTANCES FROM JOHANNESBURG BY RAIL.

To Pretoria	47 Miles.	To East London	666 Miles.
„ Delagoa Bay	398 „	„ Port Elizabeth	714 „
„ Durban	481 „	„ Cape Town	1014 „

CARRIAGE DRIVE
PARK

A U C K L A N D   P A R K

SQUARE
AVENUE
AVENUE
AVENUE
AVENUE
HIGH ST.

GALLOWAY PONY CLUB GROUND
COURSE
GRAND STAND

AGRICULTURAL SHOW
GROUND

PA

Sanitary Board's Jurisdiction Boundary

Sanitary Board's Jurisdiction Boundary

N A T I V E   L O C A T I O N

B R A M F O N T

CEMETERY

GOODS STATION

Johannesburg
Railway Station

KAFIR LOCATION   STATIONS PLEIN

COOLIE
LOCATION

BRICKFIELDS

GOODS
STATION

GasWorks

F O R D S B U R G

F E R R E
A S   T O W N

ROBINSON G.M.C.

MYFPACHT

WORCESTER G.M.C.

FERREIRA

REFERENCE.

1.	Market Hall.	41.	Bosenberg Buildings.
2.	New Post Office (Bro Long)	42.	Darnaway Buildings.
3.	Cape Govt. Railway Offices	43.	GENERAL POST and TELEGRAPH OFFICES
4.	Union Steam Ship Cos. Offices	44.	Goldreich Buildings.
5.	National Z.A.R. Bank.	45.	Royal Theatre of Varieties.
6.	Chamber of Mines	46.	Searelle's Chambers
7.	Natal Bank.	47.	Mercantile Printing Works.
8.	"The Arcade."	48.	Moore Brothers, Grocers
9.	Standard Theatre & Arcade.	49.	Castle Brewery
10.	Natal Govt. Railway Offices.	50.	Raine's Buildings
11.	Apsley & Chancellors	51.	CRITIC OFFICE and Buildings.
12.	H. Miel Auctioneer	52.	Immanuels Kerk.
13.	Stayters Buildings	53.	Delaney & Co.
14.	Papenfus Chambers	54.	Standard and Diggers News Works.
15.	Bussey Buildings	55.	Cornwell Buildings
16.	Natal Buildings & City Chambers	56.	Johannesburg Printing Company.
17.	Ecksteins.	57.	Mining Journal
18.	Exchange.	58.	Johannesburg Times Works.
19.	Robinsons Bank	59.	Albany Chambers.
20.	Post & Telegraph Office (Branch)	60.	G.R. & Ironmonger.
21.	Standard Bank.	61.	Public Hall Jeppes Town
22.	Central Buildings.	62.	Beresford Buildings.
23.	Public Library	63.	Ginsberg Chambers.
24.	Tweenes & Webster Stationers	64.	STAR OFFICE, THE ARGUS PRINTING Co.
25.	Empire Music Hall.	65.	Henwood's Arcade.
26.	Consolidated Gold Fields of South Africa.	66.	Jutas Chambers.
27.	Robinsons Buildings.	67.	Palace Buildings
28.	Roy & Chambers.	68.	ST MARYS CHURCH (ENGLISH.)
29.	Bettelheim Buildings.	69.	ST MARYS RECTORY.
30.	Nederlandsche Bank.	70.	Young Mens Christian Association.
31.	Currie Shipping Cos. Offices.	71.	Johannesburg Public School.
32.	Green's Buildings, Stamp Office.	72.	Dutch Reformed Church.
33.	Barnato Buildings.	73.	Presbyterian
34.	Mutual Buildings.	74.	Public Library
35.	T. Waddington Saddler	75.	Congregational Church.
36.	Bank of Africa	76.	Presbyterian Church.
37.	Marais Court.	77.	Congregational Church.
38.	Rand Club.	78.	Baptist Church.
39.	Aegis Buildings	79.	Chapel and Templars Hall.
40.	Zweigenhafts Buildings.	80.	Amphic Theatre.

PLAN OF
JOHANNESBURG
1896.

THE RESIDENTS' AND STRANGERS' FRIEND.

Drawn on Transfer Paper by A.E. Caplen, late Ordnance Survey of England. Transferred to Stone & Printed by ARGUS PRINTING and PUBLISHING CO.

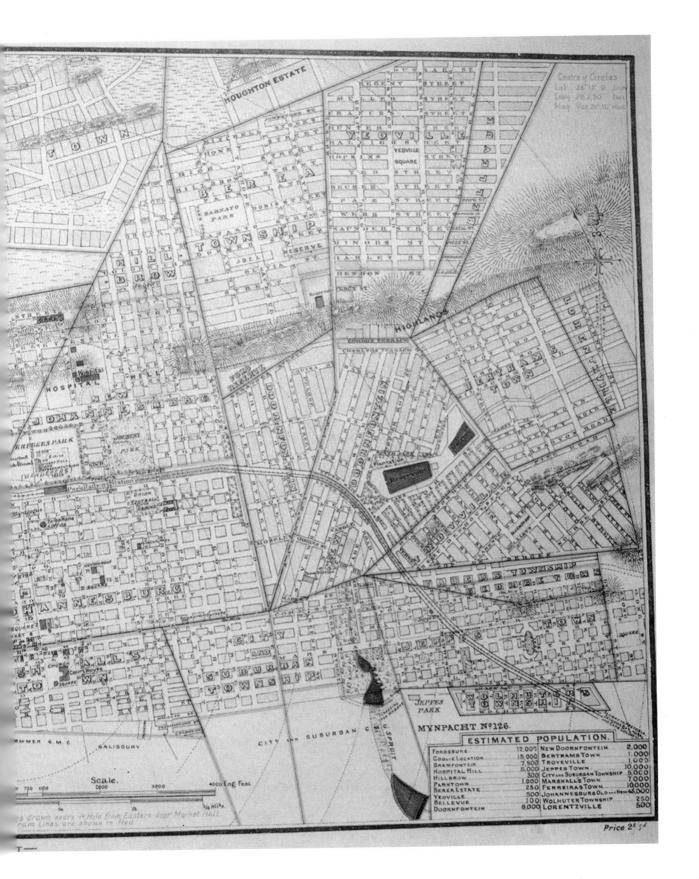

MYNPACHT N°126.

ESTIMATED POPULATION.

FORDSSURE	12,000	NEW DOORNFONTEIN	2,000
COOLIE LOCATION	15,000	BERTRAMS TOWN	1,000
BRAMFONTEIN	7,500	TROYEVILLE	1,000
HOSPITAL HILL	5,000	JEPPES TOWN	10,000
HILLBROW	300	CITY AND SUBURBAN TOWNSHIP	5,000
PARKTOWN	1,000	MARSHALLS TOWN	7,000
BEREA ESTATE	250	FERREIRAS TOWN	10,000
YEOVILLE	500	JOHANNESBURG OLD AND NEW	45,000
BELLEVUE	100	WOLHUTER TOWNSHIP	250
DOORNFONTEIN	8,000	LORENTZVILLE	500

Price 2ˢ⁶ᵈ

Scale.
0 750 1000 2000 3000 4000 Eng. Feet

...es drawn every ¼ Mile from Eastern door Market Hall
...ram Lines are shown in Red.

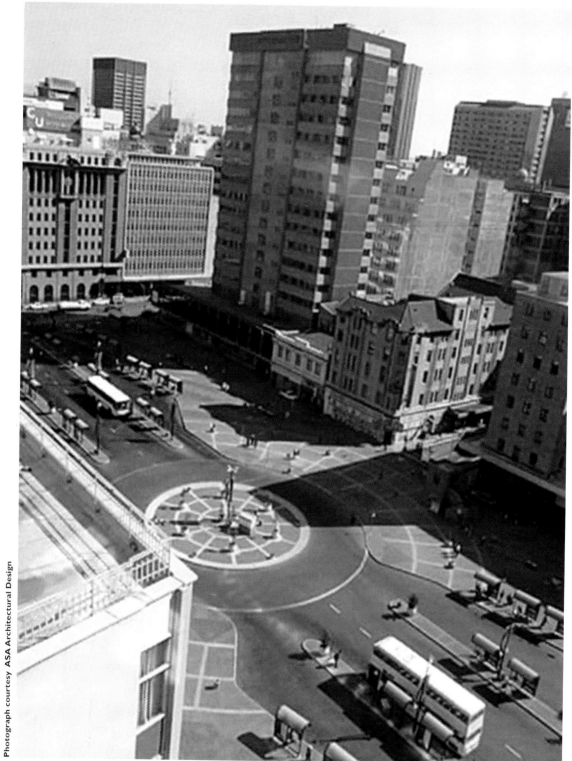

Gandhi Square

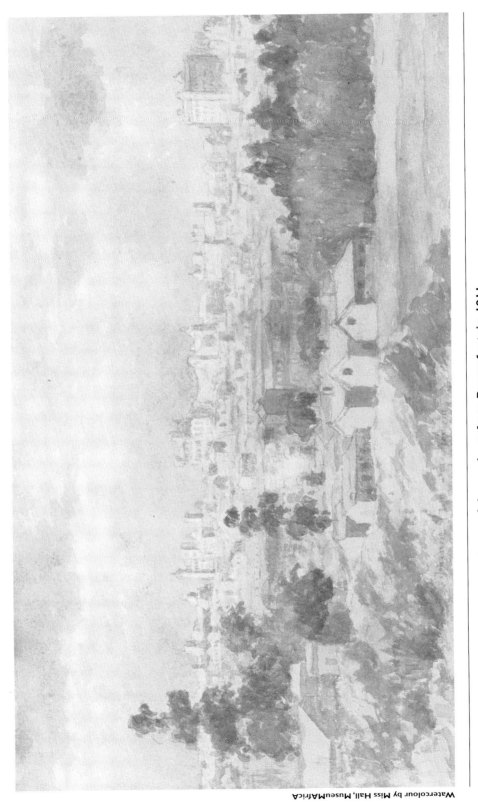

Johannesburg from Braamfontein, 1911

Watercolour by Miss Hall, MuseuMAfricA

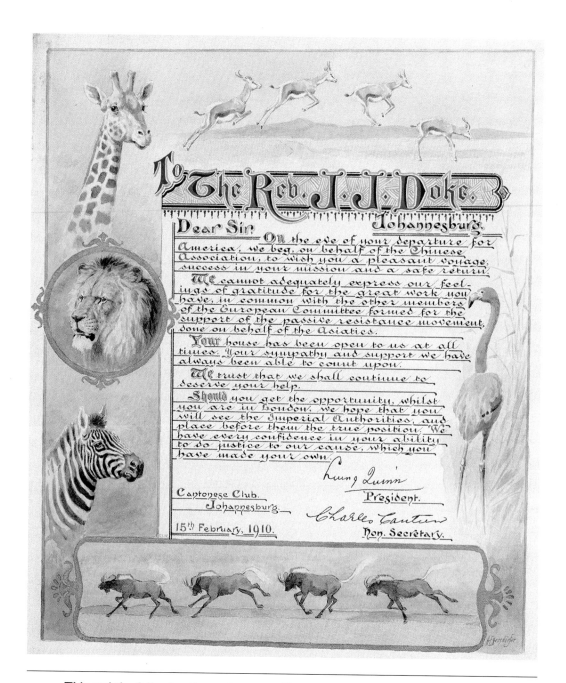

To The Rev. J. J. Doke.

Dear Sir, Johannesburg.

On the eve of your departure for America, we beg, on behalf of the Chinese Association, to wish you a pleasant voyage, success in your mission and a safe return.

We cannot adequately express our feelings of gratitude for the great work you have, in common with the other members of the European Committee formed for the support of the passive resistance movement, done on behalf of the Asiatics.

Your house has been open to us at all times. Your sympathy and support we have always been able to count upon.

We trust that we shall continue to deserve your help.

Should you get the opportunity, whilst you are in London, we hope that you will see the Imperial Authorities, and place before them the true position. We have every confidence in your ability to do justice to our cause, which you have made your own.

Leung Quinn
President.

Cantonese Club.
Johannesburg.

15th February, 1910.

Charles Canter
Hon. Secretary.

This and the following three plates are illuminated addresses presented to the Reverend Joseph Doke by community organisations

Hamidia Islamic Society

Rev. Mr. and Mrs. Doke,
                    Johannesburg.

Dear Sir, and Madam,

On behalf of the Hamidia Islamic Society, we beg to tender you our best thanks for the very warm interest you have taken in the British Indian cause in the Transvaal, and for the prompt response you have always made to our Society's appeal for help. We have no doubt that your advocacy contributed materially to the happy issue of the struggle which taxed the utmost resources of the community. The Asiatic Act specially affected the Mahomedan community in that it deliberately insulted Islam by distinguishing against Turkish Mahomedans and in favour of other Turkish Subjects. It was, therefore, natural that this Society should have made a special effort to secure the repeal of the Act, and it has been to our Society a matter of very great satisfaction that our appeal made to Mahomedans and others has been so favourably received.

We beg to remain,

Yours faithfully,

IMAM A. K. BAWAZEER,
                Chairman,

M. P. FANCY,
                Secretary.

EBRAHIM COOVADIA,
                Treasurer.

Box 6031, Johannesburg,

12th May, 1908.

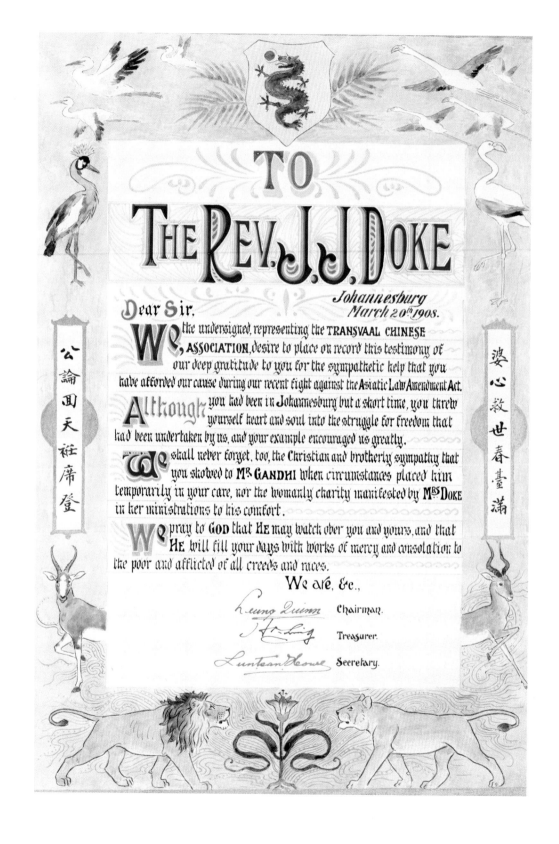

TO
THE REV. J. J. DOKE

Johannesburg
March 20th 1908.

Dear Sir,

We the undersigned, representing the TRANSVAAL CHINESE ASSOCIATION, desire to place on record this testimony of our deep gratitude to you for the sympathetic help that you have afforded our cause during our recent fight against the Asiatic Law Amendment Act.

Although you had been in Johannesburg but a short time, you threw yourself heart and soul into the struggle for freedom that had been undertaken by us, and your example encouraged us greatly.

We shall never forget, too, the Christian and brotherly sympathy that you showed to Mr GANDHI when circumstances placed him temporarily in your care, nor the womanly charity manifested by Mrs DOKE in her ministrations to his comfort.

We pray to GOD that HE may watch over you and yours, and that HE will fill your days with works of mercy and consolation to the poor and afflicted of all creeds and races.

We are, &c.,

Leung Quinn · Chairman.

H. Ling · Treasurer.

Luntsan Howe · Secretary.

公論聞天祏席登

婆心救世春臺滿

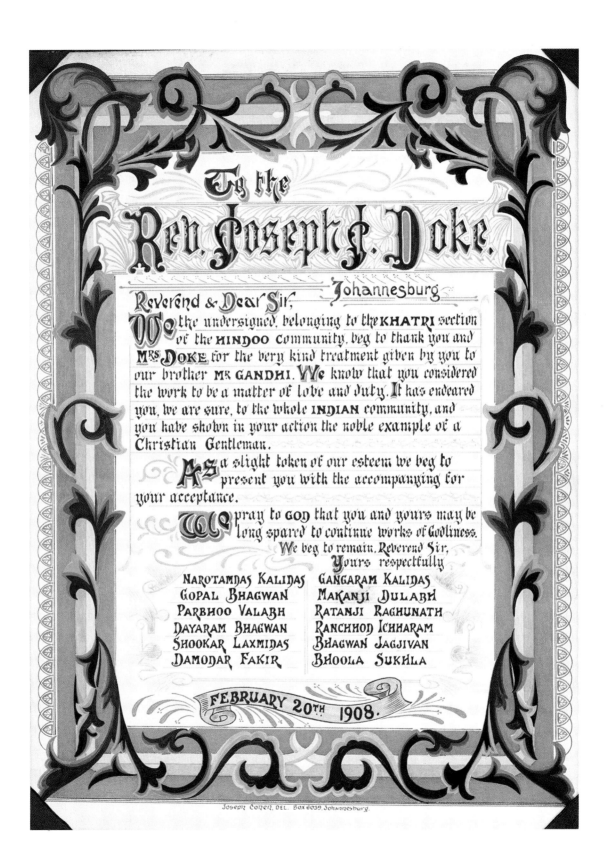

To the

Rev. Joseph J. Doke.

Johannesburg

Reverend & Dear Sir,

We the undersigned, belonging to the KHATRI section of the HINDOO community, beg to thank you and Mrs DOKE for the very kind treatment given by you to our brother MR GANDHI. We know that you considered the work to be a matter of love and duty. It has endeared you, we are sure, to the whole INDIAN community, and you have shown in your action the noble example of a Christian Gentleman.

As a slight token of our esteem we beg to present you with the accompanying for your acceptance.

We pray to GOD that you and yours may be long spared to continue works of Godliness.

We beg to remain, Reverend Sir,

Yours respectfully

NAROTAMDAS KALIDAS	GANGARAM KALIDAS
GOPAL BHAGWAN	MAKANJI DULABH
PARBHOO VALABH	RATANJI RAGHUNATH
DAYARAM BHAGWAN	RANCHHOD ICHHARAM
SHOOKAR LAXMIDAS	BHAGWAN JAGJIVAN
DAMODAR FAKIR	BHOOLA SUKHLA

FEBRUARY 20TH 1908.

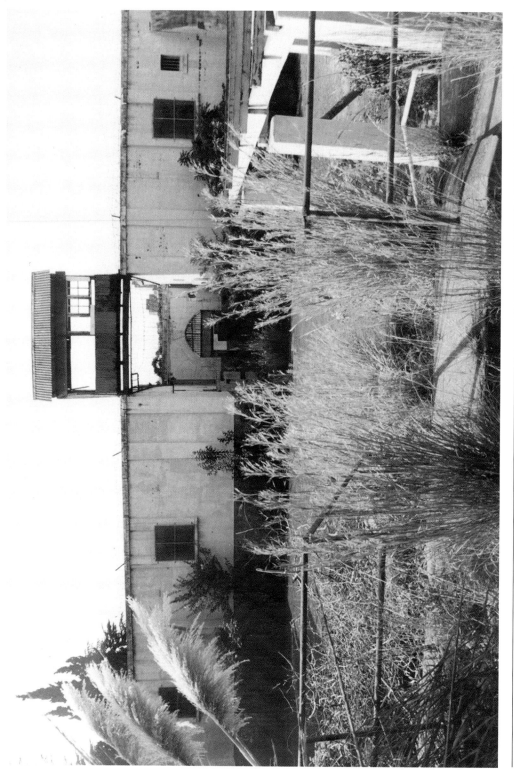

The Fort's fearsome 'Native' prison, now in disuse

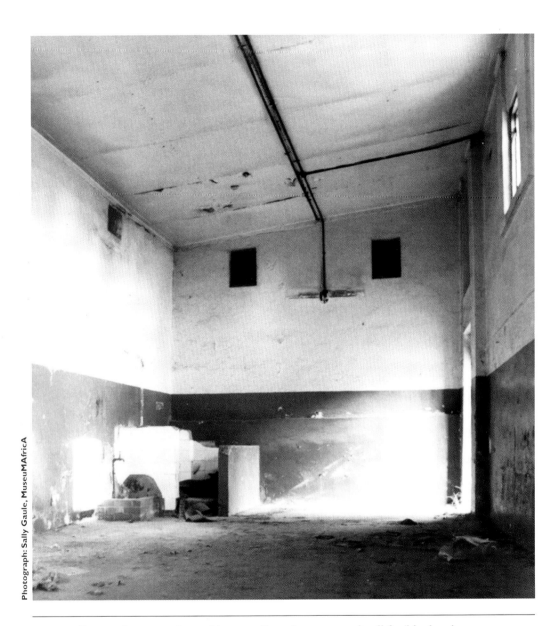

Scene of some unbearable crowding: A communal cell for black prisoners

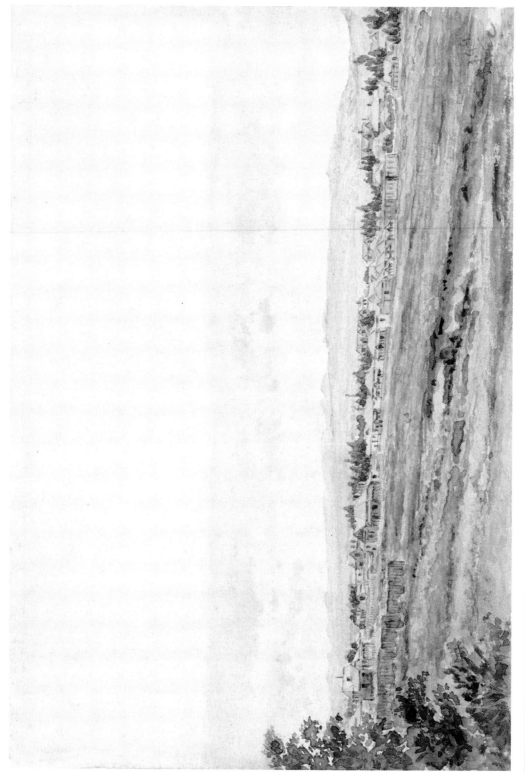

Part of Johannesburg from the bottom of Hospital Hill, 1905

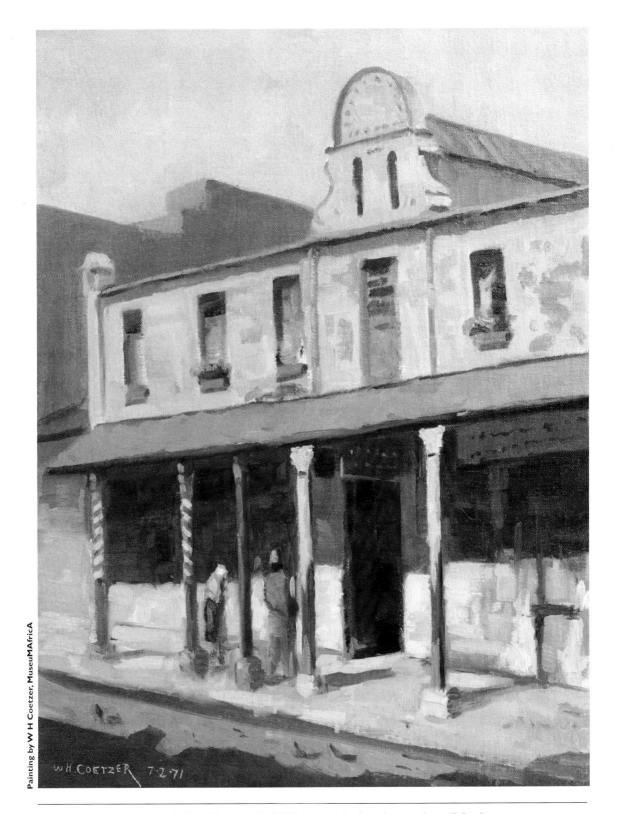

WH COETZER 7-2-71

The Gaiety Theatre in 1971, a year before it was demolished

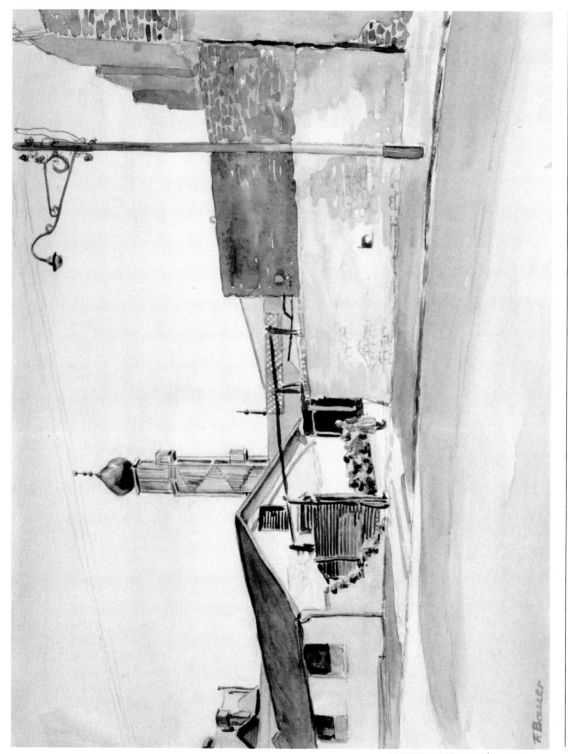

Newtown with a view of the minaret of the Hamidia Mosque

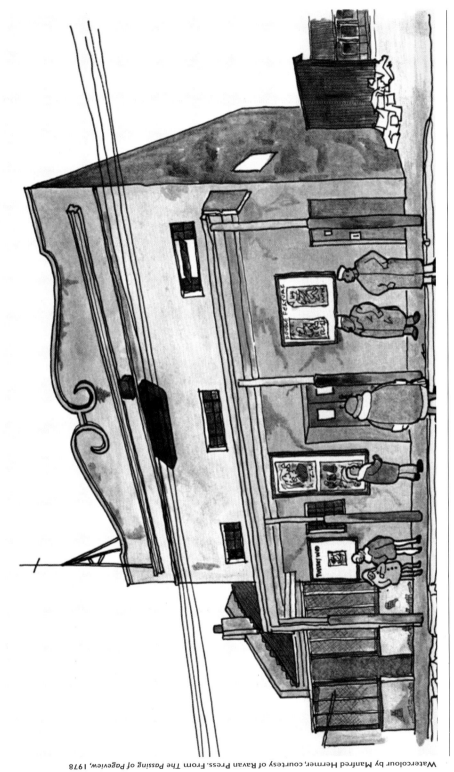

Pageview's Taj Cinema, once a centre of political activity known as the Hamidia Hall

Watercolour by Manfred Hermer, courtesy of Ravan Press. From *The Passing of Pageview*, 1978

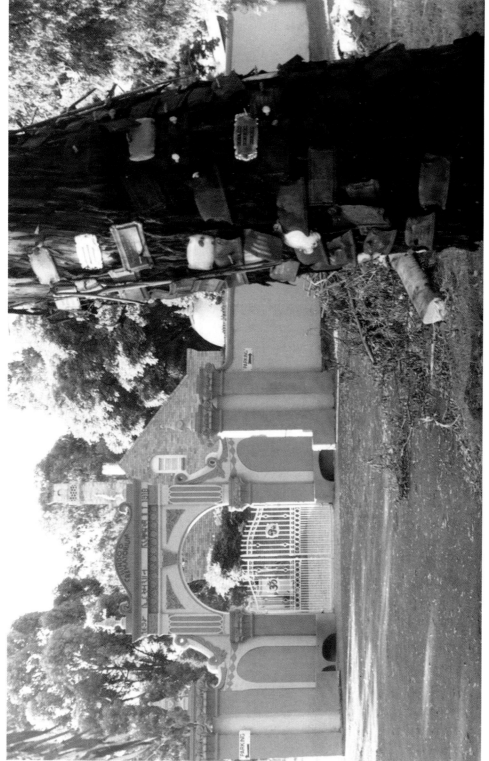

Entrance to the crematorium. Tin plates from coffins are nailed to the tree in the foreground

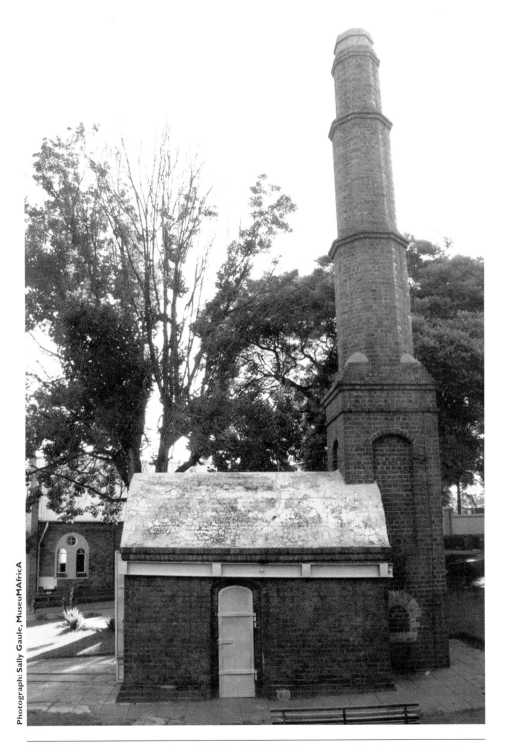

The Hindu Crematorium built in 1918 in Brixton was the first brick-built
crematorium in the southern hemisphere

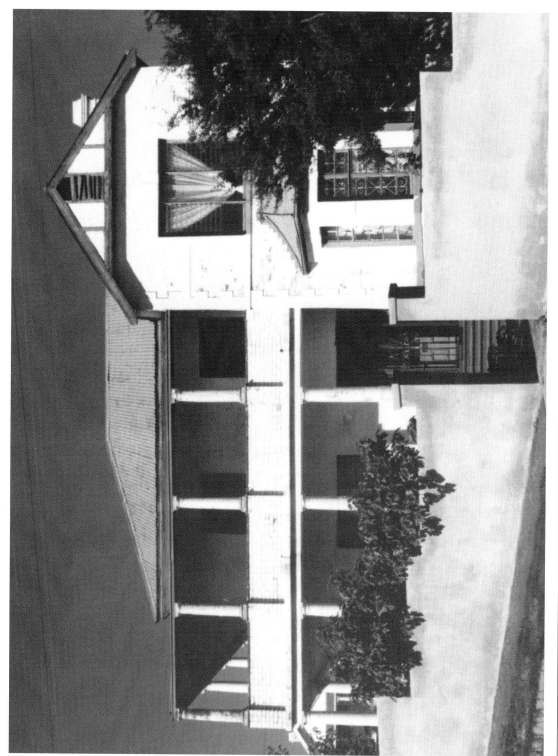

Troyeville's Gandhi house as it looks today

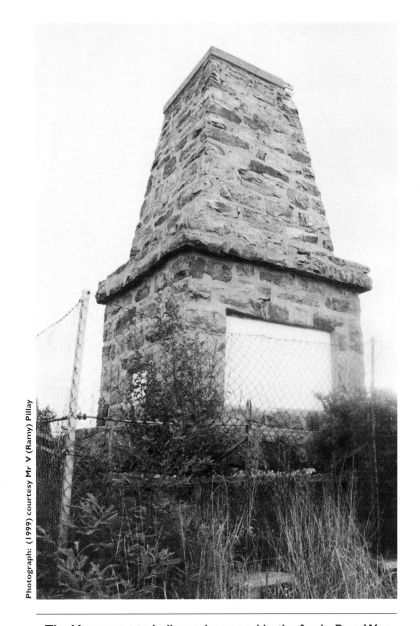

The Monument to Indians who served in the Anglo-Boer War

'The monument stands as a reminder of
the sacrifice of men who came thousands
of miles to serve a cause, but also of those
others who pleaded with astonishing persistance to
be allowed to shoulder their share of the danger and discomfort'

Knox and Gutsche

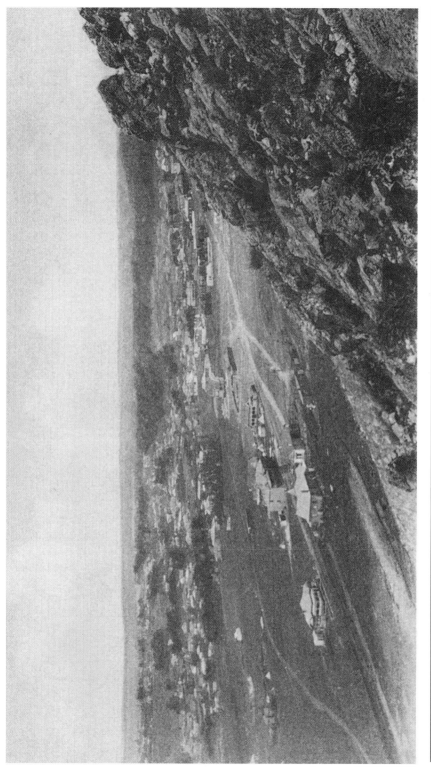

Johannesburg from Bellevue East, circa 1905